Stretching for Health & Performance

The Complete Handbook for All Ages & Fitness Levels

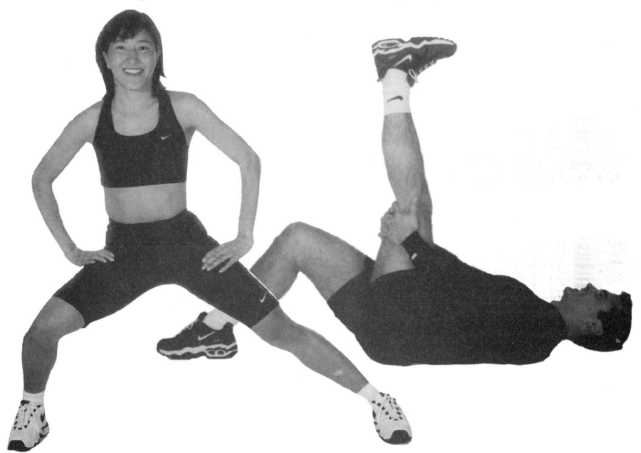

Dr. Christopher A. Oswald &
Dr. Stanley N. Bacso

Illustrations by Jason Branicky

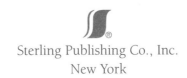

Sterling Publishing Co., Inc.
New York

Library of Congress Cataloging-in-Publication Data Available

10   9   8   7   6

Published by Sterling Publishing Co., Inc.
387 Park Avenue South, New York, NY 10016
Distributed in Canada by Sterling Publishing
c/o Canadian Manda Group, One Atlantic Avenue, Suite 105
Toronto, Ontario, Canada M6K 3E7
Distributed in Great Britain by Chrysalis Books Group PLC
The Chrysalis Building, Bramley Road, London W10 6SP, England
Distributed in Australia by Capricorn Link (Australia) Pty. Ltd.
P.O. Box 704, Windsor, NSW 2756, Australia

Manufactured in the United States of America

Sterling ISBN 0-8069-0985-4

Contents

Foreword   4

Acknowledgments   4

Chapter 1
Introduction   5

Chapter 2
The Fundamentals of Stretching   7

Chapter 3
Stretching for All Ages   13

Chapter 4
Calcium & Magnesium: Muscle
Fibers & Stretching   20

Chapter 5
Understanding Your Body &
Its Limits   23

Chapter 6
Six Rules to Stretching   26

Chapter 7
The Basic Stretches & Their
Anatomy   28

Chapter 8
The Daily Shower Routine   63

Chapter 9
Dangerous & Harmful
Movements   67

Chapter 10
Stretches for Specific Sports   75

Chapter 11
Stretching for Injury Rehabilitation
& Pain Syndromes   127

Chapter 12
Stretches for Specific
Occupations   150

Chapter 13
Household Activities: Stretches &
Postures   159

Chapter 14
Stretching for Pregnancy &
Delivery   172

Chapter 15
Exercises for the Abdomen &
Low Back   184

Index   190

About the Authors   192

F o r e w o r d

It is a pleasure for me to endorse *Stretching for Fitness, Health & Performance*. There is a wealth of conflicting and incomplete information which has flooded the marketplace in the last few years regarding health enhancement through stretching, exercise, and nutrition. Having witnessed a serious shortcoming in education regarding safe and effective stretching methods for the general public, these authors have developed this user-friendly manual that can teach everyone the key concepts of stretching. My evaluation of the work finds it not only technically sound, but completely understandable for anyone who wishes to stretch for health. This book should help the young and old, the active and inactive as well as prevent injuries at work, play, or exercise.

Dr. Douglas Pooley
President-Canadian Chiropractic Association

As practitioners, we are frequently asked by patients for advice on specific exercise programs or suitable reading material on stretching. Inevitably, we refer to the one or two exercise reference manuals on our shelf to put together a program, which includes separate information sheets on what to do and not do as well as home treatment protocols. This process is often very time consuming. Dr. Oswald and Mr. Bacso have done an excellent job in presenting a text that will address all the above needs. Their text provides patients with a basic understanding of anatomy, body mechanics, and the principles of stretching that are emphasized in their application to specific sports and daily life activities. Geared towards all ages and activity levels, this text will serve both the practitioner and the public extremely well.

Silvano A. Mior, DC, FCCS(C)
Dean of Graduate Studies and Research
Canadian Memorial Chiropractic College

A c k n o w l e d g m e n t s

We would like to thank everyone who was instrumental in the creation of this book. We are deeply grateful to all, particularly the following for their suggestions, time, insight, and contributions: Bob Wilkenson, Marni Grossman and her photography assistants Jamie, Brian, and Joseph; Rick Diamond, Jay Grossman, Charles Nurnberg, John Woodside, Karen Nelson, Rhonda Feduck, Lisa Morante, Shauna Parr, Dr. Paul Carey, Alan Kerslake, Karen Reid, Suzanne Merrett, Clare Ollerhead, Dr. Donald Sutherland, Cynthia MacKenzie, Ed Bergman, John Waddell, Mark Hamilton, Stephen R. Bacso, Dr. Doug Pooley, Dr. Sil Mior, Dr. Jerry Grod, Dr. Brian Hands, Catherine Fournier, Sandy Goss, David Chapman-Smith, Neil Skinner, Catherine Bruder, Jason Branicky, Dennis Mills, Cynthia Baker, Chris Hedges, Dan Hill, Dr. Chris Bardwell, Brian and Ginny Kerslake, Janice Hollett, Craig Alexander, Morey and Ephram Chaplick, Larry Wasser, David Harmes, Michelle Lynch, Erin Hurst; Karl, Adrienne, and Eddie of Straub sporting goods; Mark Porter and the Cricket Club, Bill Ford, Liz MacDonald, Patrick McGee, Laura Newland, Kwame Addo, Edna Chu, Shelia Morrow-Oswald, Madison Oswald, Paul Rowan, Cathy Donkersley, Dr. Blair Lewis, Joshua Samuel, Peter Adams, and Dr. Ron and Dianna Oswald.

Introduction

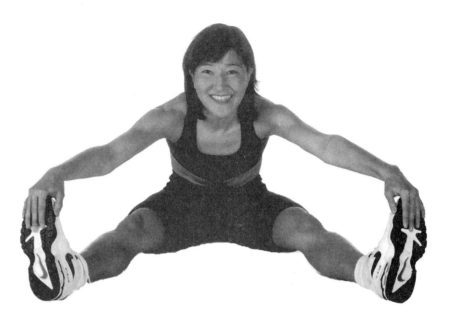

*T*his user-friendly manual was specifically designed to discuss and show both the basic and advanced concepts that underlie the need to stretch for optimal health and performance in everything that you do. From a chiropractic perspective and 18 years of experience in the science and art of stretching, we have found that stretching safely and effectively can happen only when you combine the fields of mechanics, neurology, physiology, and athletics. Therefore, stretching is seen as an integral part of rehabilitation in musculoskeletal injuries and developmental problems. It is also a tremendously cost effective method of preventing injuries, maintaining mobility, reducing stress, and enhancing performance and the quality of life.

Although there are numerous books on stretching, some lack the understanding behind the stretching while others lack the practical information and application of it. Most do not have the complete information of both areas to make stretching truly effective. This is why the general population is merely going through the motions when it comes to stretching. As a result, many people make mistakes and experience serious injuries by overstretching, poor posture, and a lack of understanding how the body works.

For example, it is distressing to read some of the new yoga books around today. The ancient art and philosophy of yoga is making a modern-day comeback by using such terms as power, total strength, body sculpting, yogarobics, etc. But yoga, by definition, means enlightenment and self-realization. It employs powerful breathing techniques and a wide range of postures/positions to achieve relaxation or enlightenment.

Although we, as scientists, agree that breathing

is an essential means of relaxation, that the *chakras*, or the seven energy centers of the body, are in close proximity with important nerve bundles, and that the body is more flexible when properly warmed up, it must be made clear that yoga was not designed to make you more flexible; it was designed to help you seek "inner peace." Therefore, the terms "stretching" and "yoga" should not be used interchangeably. In fact, it is easy for the untrained eye to see from looking at the many positions employed in yoga that they are not designed to be gentle and safe for everyone of any age group. They are, for the majority, strenuous on the joints, muscles, ligaments, etc.

This manual, with the most current understanding of bones, joints, muscles, ligaments, nerves, and blood supply, was created to help facilitate flexibility, movement, and fitness. By stretching safely, it is easy to achieve relaxation and perhaps greater self-awareness. We will teach you how to pay attention to your various body parts and help you understand your capabilities and limitations. Perhaps you can become enlightened, but we feel that you first must find your toes before you find your aura.

This manual presents a thorough picture of the art, science, and philosophy of stretching from books, manuals, scientific journals, and guides on stretching in the last 15 years. There are also numerous analogies, facts, and examples to help you understand stretching. All of the routines in this book can be done by anyone from any age group, whether or not you are under medical care. They are especially good for maintaining health, flexibility, and fitness. Since every human body has its individual strengths and weaknesses, we suggest that you ask your chiropractor or physician to help you understand which stretches are best for you.

The first part of this manual discusses the science and fundamentals of stretching, and presents reasons why all age groups should stretch. The remaining chapters demonstrate, with photos, how to stretch properly and move every muscle in the human body. To ensure effective teaching, we have included detailed pictures of the muscle being stretched along with the actual stretch (see Chapter 7). If you can visualize the direction of the muscle fibers and understand the job of a particular muscle, then you can maximize your ability to stretch effectively and successfully. Chapter 9 may surprise you by explaining why some stretches and exercises that you may have been performing for years are actually not good for you.

You will also find appropriate warm-up and cool-down routines for all types of sports, stretching routines for the different stages of pregnancy, proper posture guidelines and stretching routines for many household chores and work duties, and stretch programs for people that suffer from various disorders and conditions, ranging from migraine headaches to tennis elbow.

We have thoroughly examined *all* types of stretching and have included only the ones that have been tested to be safe. We hope that this instructional manual helps add years to your life and life to your years!

The Fundamentals of Stretching

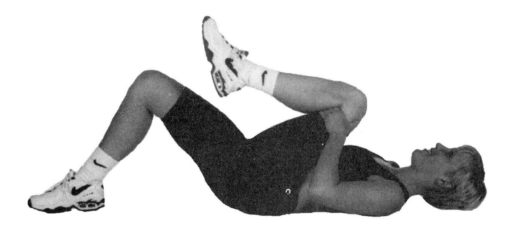

*M*obility and pain-free movement of the muscles are critical factors in how you live your life. When you suffer from pain or discomfort, it can hinder your daily activities. Stretching can facilitate mobility, improve muscle mechanics, and allow you greater opportunities every day. To master the basics of stretching, you need to understand its fundamental concepts.

DEFINITION AND GOAL OF STRETCHING

A stretch is a specific position sustained to increase and maintain the length of a muscle or a muscle group. It lengthens tendons, warms up ligaments, and prepares joints for work. As a result, there is:

1. Additional flexibility throughout the body.
2. Decreased tightness or stiffness.
3. Improved awareness of muscles and their capabilities during any daily activity or sport.
4. Increased coordination and agility in daily or recreational activities.
5. Decreased blood pressure and a "fit" cardiovascular system.
6. Enhanced circulation, which provides muscles with oxygen and other nutrients for the support structures of the human frame.
7. Quicker removal of waste products (lactic acid, carbon dioxide, nitrogen, cellular metabolites) from the muscles.
8. Reduced pressure on joint cartilage and spinal discs, which reduces the arthritic wear-and-tear process (osteoarthritis or degenerative disc disease).

9. Reduced inflammation and pain of the joints often seen in numerous types of arthritic conditions (rheumatoid arthritis, gout, Reiter's syndrome).

10. Less stress on the nervous system.

11. Facilitation of overall health and sense of well-being.

FLEXIBILITY VS. STRETCHING

Flexibility means having the freedom to move. It is a major part of everything you do. By following a specific routine geared to your physical make-up, stretching dramatically improves flexibility. This added mobility is critical because even the easiest tasks require movement: rising out of bed in the morning, stepping into the tub or shower, reaching into a cupboard/closet, leaning over and tying your shoes, lifting a baby out of a crib, getting something from a car trunk, working at a job, climbing up the stairs, and exercising safely and effectively.

As a result, stretching can be considered even more important than exercising. However, stretching coupled with exercise is the key to lifelong health and well-being.

EXERCISE VS. STRETCHING

Exercise is a specific work or activity geared towards:

1. Strengthening muscles.

2. Improving cardiovascular function.

3. Strengthening the immune system.

4. Stimulating body chemicals (epinephrine, endorphin).

5. Reducing stress.

6. Rehabilitating from injury.

7. Improving ability and stamina for additional work or play.

Since exercise is a form of work, the human frame requires preparation in order to perform work safely. Stretching helps you prepare for any activity by altering your muscle resilience or tone. It should be done both before and after work or exercise. Stretching before (as part of a warm-up) prepares tissues for work, and stretching after (cool-down) helps tissues recover from the strain or stress of the work/exercise. Examples of work/exercise includes:

1. Using the treadmill, walking, jogging, weight lifting, and all other sports (see Chapter 10).

2. Household activities like vacuuming, cleaning, raking, moving, and gardening (see Chapter 13).

3. Job requirements for accountants, doctors, lawyers, restaurant workers, students, musicians, etc. (see Chapter 12).

WHAT HAPPENS IN A STRETCH?

All the stretches in this manual are static stretches, which are controlled and slow. In a static stretch, as you stretch a muscle in a slow and gentle fashion, you increase its tension. In a few milliseconds, the spinal cord reflexively tells the muscle to shorten in order to protect the muscle from being overstretched. It takes 6–10 seconds for the brain and spinal cord to perceive that the stretch is safe and, suddenly, the mild pulling sensation you feel of the muscle shortening to resist the stretch is gone. It is in the next 20–24 seconds that the stretch has the beneficial effects. That is why a stretch must be held for at least 30 seconds.

A good rule to follow is that if you feel the uncomfortable stretching sensation for more than 10 seconds, you are stretching *too far* and *too fast*.

You should ease off slightly until the sensation is gone and then hold for 30 seconds (see Chapter 6 for the Six Rules to Stretching).

It is important that you do *not* bounce when you stretch. This kind of stretching, known as a ballistic stretch, creates more than double the amount of tension as compared to a static stretch. Even though it is done in many aerobic classes and workout videos, it may actually cause nerve damage and muscle-fiber tearing. It also does not improve flexibility.

WHEN SHOULD YOU STRETCH?

Ideally, stretching should be done when the body is warm. That way, there is sufficient blood flow carrying important minerals, such as calcium and magnesium (see Chapter 4), throughout the tissues before you begin to stretch. Optimum muscular relaxation is also the key to effective stretching. Mid-morning, after lunch, and early evening are excellent times to stretch, since the body has already been moving around and has the required nutrients supplied (assuming from a proper diet). Realistically though, most individuals cannot stop in the middle of the day to engage in "lengthy" stretch routines, nor will they take time in the evening to stretch, because they are tired or have other commitments. It is with this thought in mind that we developed the shower stretch routine.

In the Shower

Since most people shower daily, it is a good place to incorporate stretching. Most people do not mind spending an extra 5 to 10 minutes in a warm shower to do something good for their bodies. If you bathe instead of shower, you can stretch in the living room or bedroom in the morning after you bathe.

A morning stretch prepares the muscles and the human frame for the daily stressors encountered. It also significantly reduces the chance of injury or the recurrence of pain from previous injuries. The shower/morning stretch routine is easy to follow and remember (see Chapter 8). But if you cannot remember, you can always hang our laminated program in the shower.

Warming Up

Wherever you do your stretching, you must perform some minimal movement first. In the shower, this can be washing your body. Elsewhere, it can be marching in place, riding a stationary bike, or anything that gets the blood flowing without causing strain. A warm-up consists of 2–5 minutes of movement *plus* a stretching routine. The goal is to get the blood flowing *without* challenging the body to new heights! The average person and professional athlete will often injure themselves if they engage in too vigorous movements prior to stretching. Their "cold" muscles, tendons, and ligaments are not prepared to deal with the sudden onset of strain, which can cause ankle sprains, pinched spinal nerves, or ruptured Achilles tendons.

The warm-up and stretch routine should consist of 15–20% of the total workout time. For example, if you exercise for 60 minutes, you need 9–12 minutes of warm-up.

Cooling Down

After every activity, especially taxing ones, you should do a cool-down stretch routine, similar to the warm-up stretch, to relax the muscles that were just exercised. This helps eliminate the metabolic build-up of waste, such as lactic acid, nitrogen, and carbon dioxide, from the muscles to enhance muscle repair and recovery. Otherwise, the metabolic waste will cause muscle stiffness, which affects the movement of the joints.

By cooling down, you will help reduce the muscle soreness that may occur after a particularly stressful activity as well as prevent blood pooling, dizziness, heart palpitation, and nausea. If you incorporate deep abdominal breathing during the cool-down, you will increase the cellular waste removal even more.

A cool-down should consist of 5–15% of the total workout time. For example, if you exercise for 60 minutes, you need 3–9 minutes of cooling down. Ideally, if you stretch during your exercise (e.g., during weight-lifting sets, you stretch the muscle that you are training for 30 seconds after each set), it will make your cool-down much more time efficient.

THE NEED FOR STRETCHING

On the Job

If you are in a heavy-lifting or excessive-sitting job (the two most common causes of low back pain and repetitive strain injuries in North America), you should do a brief stretch routine every hour for 2–3 minutes. This, in conjunction with a morning stretch routine, will help you to cope with specific problem areas better and

allow you to keep working at top efficiency. It will also allow you to enjoy all your recreational activities.

If your job requires periods of lifting then resting, it is beneficial to apply an intermittent stretch routine best suited for the type of strain you undergo (see Chapter 12: Stretches for Specific Occupations). Doing this before the start of each lifting period will markedly reduce injury.

If your job requires you to sit or stand for a long period of time, you are then engaging in a static position for an excessive amount of time. As a result, stiffness can occur in various parts of the body. To understand why this happens, let's examine the result of static work.

The diagram below shows the work done by an arm in relaxation, static (non-moving) work, and dynamic (moving) work. The columns underneath each diagram represent the amount of blood flow to the muscles. Under each diagram, the left column is the blood flow required by the muscle, and the right column is the blood supply or fuel actually received.

The picture on the left shows that when a

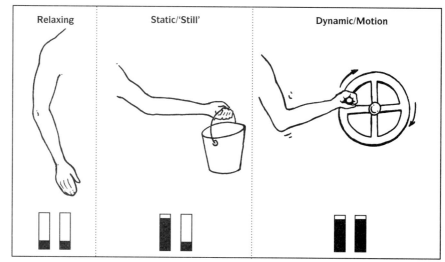

muscle is relaxed, it requires little fuel. The picture on the right shows that when a muscle is moving properly, the blood flow requirements are maintained. However, when a muscle is held in one position without moving (center picture), the fuel demand of the muscle does not equal the actual flow it receives. This condition is called static muscle loading, and it is caused by long periods of muscle contraction or shortening from some types of postures. The reduced blood flow means less oxygen or fuel supply to the muscle. As a result, metabolic waste products, such as lactic acid, are created and muscular fatigue occurs. This leads to various types of pain, such as headaches, shoulder stiffness, or low back pain, which are commonly suffered from repetitive stress injuries at stationary jobs (see Chapter 12).

It takes 1 minute working at a moderate level of intensity, or 4 minutes at a mild level of intensity, to produce muscle fatigue symptoms.

Doing Housework

Compared to heavy weight-lifting or intense aerobics, working around the house may not seem like an overly stressful task. However, the culmination of small stresses and strain—from gardening, vacuuming, raking to lifting—can lead to serious spinal misalignments, muscle strains, and pain if precautionary measures, such as stretching, are neglected. Many people do not regard housework as taxing. This is not true! Household chores can produce enough stress to injure the body if it is not prepared for work. Vacuuming,

raking, and shoveling snow produce the worst and most frequent injuries (see Chapter 13).

Emotional Stress

Besides the physical stress of work, we should not forget the emotional stress that occasionally affects us. If you had a particularly stressful day, you should do a basic "head to toe" stretch routine to help you relax and get a proper night's sleep. Without proper sleep, you cannot think as clearly, and the stress you experience is multiplied. As a result, you can become more irritable, angry, and frustrated. If sleep deprivation continues, you can experience burnout, chronic fatigue, insomnia, pain, and, at worst, a complete nervous breakdown.

A perfect example is postpartum depression, or "post-delivery blues," which is significantly exacerbated by lack of sleep. Stretching can be an important component in alleviating the stress and helping the body to recover (see Chapter 14).

1–2% of Your Day

Although it may seem that some form of stretching should be done all the time, nothing could be further from the truth. Surprisingly, little stretching time is required to make noticeable gains. An average morning stretch routine in the shower takes about 5–10 minutes and produces great results. At work, you may stretch specific tight muscles two to four times a day for 2 minutes (total of 4–8 minutes). If you exercise three times a week for an hour each time, you would warm up with 10 minutes of stretching and cool down for 5 minutes (total of 15 minutes).

Let's say that 1 or 2 days a week you may be in a particularly stressful state and, consequently, stretch for 10–15 minutes. On average then, you might stretch about 25 minutes a day. That constitutes approximately 1–2% of your day!

Since stretching is a passive activity, it should be considered relaxing as opposed to something that requires effort. Remember, exercise is work, stretching is *not*. You can stretch while sitting or lying in front of the television. Compare this to the average person who watches television for over 2 hours a day, or 8% of the day. If you only stretched while watching television, you would quickly rise to an expert level of flexibility. Even if you were to stretch only during the commercials, you would attain a good level of flexibility in a very short time.

But you should have fun with stretching. Let it be a form of meditation. Use it to relax, unwind, contemplate, get away from the world for a few minutes, or plan your next day. It can be both physically and psychologically rewarding.

Stretch Break

Tilt right ear toward right shoulder.

Hold for 30 seconds (about three to five deep breaths).

Feel a gentle pull on the side-neck muscles.

Breathe normally; repeat on the other side.

Stretching for All Ages

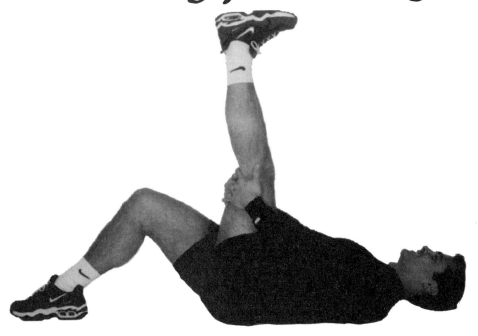

INFANTS

Birth has been said to be the most traumatic experience in one's life, but its physical and emotional stresses cannot be fully understood. The infancy stage has always caused a great deal of difficulty for health practitioners and patients because:

1. Most authorities, until recently, felt that babies were resilient (i.e., if they fell, they would bounce right back);

2. Most infants cannot communicate what they are feeling or where they feel discomfort.

Although there is still debate today by pediatric physicians and psychologists over these two views, much research has been recently done to help us better appreciate the stresses to the infant.

In childbirth, the emotional and mental stressors include the shock of leaving a dark, warm, fluid-filled, quiet environment and arriving in a hospital room full of people, noises, bright lights, etc. The social stressors include the infant's realization that it is no longer the only person in the world. Although the emotional, mental, and social stresses are hard to quantify, the physical stressors are easier to measure. During natural childbirth, forces in excess of 90 lbs. per square inch are applied in a twisting and pulling direction to a newborn's head, neck, and shoulders, particularly when forceps or vacuums are used. Ultimately, brain stem damage or, more commonly, minor injuries (such as neck nerve and muscle-tissue failure), which develop later in life, can occur.

Childbirth Injuries

A 1986 study showed that 2.5 of 1000 childbirth injuries are to the brachial plexus, a bundle of nerves that exit the spinal cord from the lower neck region and connect to the neck, arms, hands, chest and shoulders. As a result, the infant can have the following symptoms:

1. Wryneck, or congenital toricollis, in which the infant holds its head to one side. This is often caused by an overstretching of the front of the neck.
2. Erb's palsy, in which the infant holds the arms close to the body with elbows straight, wrists flexed into a "waiter's tip" position, and palms facing backward. The damage here is usually to the neck nerve roots that enter the upper limb from the lower neck area.
3. Klumpke's palsy, in which the infant's elbow and hand are set in a claw-like hand position. This is the result of compression of the brachial plexus.

A traumatic birth process can also result in spinal joint blockages, or damage to the spinal bones (vertebrae). Since the nerve structures of the spinal cord are not elastic (like muscles and ligaments), they are more easily damaged from twisting forces. Spinal joint problems can have numerous other far-reaching effects, including colic, ear infections, tonsillitis, eating disorders, weakened immune system, and sleeping disorders. Damage to the vertebrae and nerves may prevent normal bone growth or may even lead to asymmetries, such as scoliosis. Although there is no definitive data on the extent of birth trauma's effect on an individual's adult life, evidence suggests that it is more far-reaching than previously thought.

More common than major birth-process traumas are the minor effects, which over a prolonged period of time can lead to structural and functional problems, such as a strained neck. If left untreated, which is usually what happens, they can become difficult to treat in later years.

On the brighter side, there are alternative methods of health care and health professionals who view infant injury as significant and "real." For example, chiropractic literature has reported one of the largest and most successful studies for the treatment of infantile colic through stretching.

Colic is a spasmodic, cramplike pain in the abdomen. The otherwise healthy and thriving young infant cries persistently and often violently. It is different from normal crying because the distress does not stop when the infant's physiological needs are met (i.e., feeding, sleeping). Studies show that gently stretching (or manipulating) the vertebral column of the infant's spine can safely and effectively treat most colic cases.

Stretching for Infants

What about the normal, healthy baby that sits in a car seat, perhaps for hours? It needs stretching of tight muscles in order to continue developing properly. Otherwise, this may lead to slouching, and back and neck problems later on. Stiff muscles can begin in infancy. These techniques will keep your child more comfortable, particularly because they will set a good posture, which helps reduce gas and upset stomach—the most common complaints from new parents. At the same time, they will help prevent poor muscle conditions that can hinder normal growth and contribute to future problems (see next page).

CHILDREN

Some authorities feel that many complaints from children are insignificant and inconsequential. Many others feel that the child is being insolent

HOW TO IMPROVE INFANT FLEXIBILITY AND COMFORT

1. Place a 1-inch thick small pillow or rolled towel in the car seat to give the child some support to the low back area. Have it 3 inches above the waist.

2. Lift the child under the arms a few times a day and allow the spine and legs to hang and stretch out. Hold for 20–30 seconds.

3. Lay the child on its back and take a gentle hold of the shin bones of both legs. Help the child to completely straighten the knee of one leg and then bend it while straightening the other, much like riding a bike. Do this twice a day for 5 minutes. Hold for 20–30 seconds in each position.

or will simply grow out of the problem. We feel that this view is not only irresponsible, but also dangerous.

"As the twig is bent, so grows the tree."

Musculoskeletal problems that have occurred in childhood develop into or create other problems as life progresses. These problems might have been prevented if the child had been taken to an appropriate doctor earlier.

Since 80% of adults experience low back pain, our study shows that problems that begin early in life *only* get worse in time if ignored. That is why preventative stretching and lifestyle adjustments are essential. Parents, teachers, and doctors should focus on:

1. Educating children on stretching, exercise, health, lifestyle, anatomy, and posture.

2. Modifying or changing the sitting habits of children. This is usually a long-term strategy starting in the elementary school years.

Oswald Survey (1992)

1. 53% of junior/senior kindergarten children suffered headaches; 47% experienced low back pain (LBP).

2. 93% of Grade 1 pupils suffered headaches; 39% experienced LBP.

3. 83% of Grade 4 pupils suffered headaches; 43% experienced LBP.

Growing Pains

More often than not you inherit, not necessarily a disease or pain syndrome, but the tendency to develop a particular pain. What you do, or don't do, contributes to the presence or absence of certain problems. For example, "growing pains" is the term often used to describe pain in the shins or knees in children at the time of accelerated growth. Growing pains can often last from 6 months to 3 years. They can affect one, or both, legs and persist even when growing has subsided. It has been assumed that the muscles of the legs were not growing fast enough to keep up with the underlying bones, which in turn leads to a tension in the muscle tendon where it attaches to the bone, usually below the knee cap.

However, if the pain persists after growth slows down or stops:

1. How can the pain be from growing?

2. If the pain occurs on one side only, how can it be growing pains when the body grows relatively evenly on both sides?

Case Study:

M.F., a 14-year-old boy, had growing pains in the knees for 2 years. He saw numerous doctors with no success. After a thorough history, knee examination, low back examination, and X-ray, a low back problem was discovered to be responsible for the sharp leg pains. Stretches were given and the problem was resolved within 3–4 weeks. To date, 7 years later, he has not had a recurrence of leg/knee pain.

HOW TO IMPROVE A CHILD'S GROWING PAINS

1. Stretch the hamstring, quadriceps, and groin muscles.

2. Apply ice packs to the knees for 10 minutes at a time at least three to five times a day.

3. Consult a chiropractor who will "correct" the spine, if necessary.

4. Consult an orthopedic surgeon if the problem persists after conservative treatment.

Stretching for Children

This stretch routine can be done in the morning. Keep it fun. Keep it simple. Do not worry if they make up their own stretches. It is important that they develop an interest in stretching at this stage of life.

It will likely be difficult to get any child to hold each stretch for 30 seconds, breathe, and, above all, do it in perfect form. Simply do your best to direct them. Let them try to copy you doing your routine.

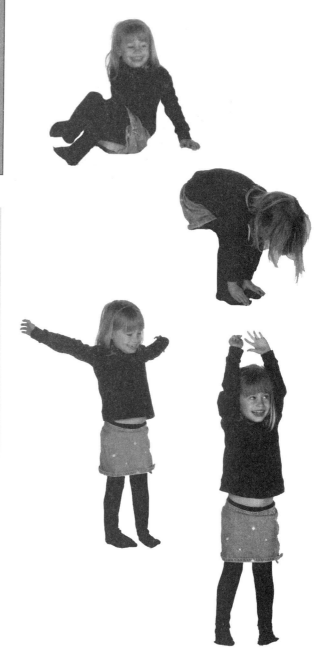

ADOLESCENTS

Teenagers are prone to posture-related stress. Slouching in chairs, carrying heavy bags or knapsacks over one shoulder, playing school sports without adequate preparation, and a general lack of postural awareness and importance are the main causes. At this stage of their lives, adolescents often suffer from static muscle loading (see p. 10) and significant body aches and pains.

How to Carry School Supplies Properly

The photo on the left is the ideal way to carry school supplies. By keeping the spine aligned, the pelvis and shoulders are level. If your posture is like the photo in the middle or on the right, there is significant strain on the human frame. Carrying your supplies on the right side and then switching to the left will not balance the load and

negate potential problems. You will simply strain both shoulders independently.

Since the average adolescent can carry some 20–30 lbs. of books and supplies in a knapsack to school daily, many experience pain, particularly around the neck and shoulders. This can lead to headaches and problems in concentrating, which cause problems in learning.

HOW TO IMPROVE ADOLESCENT FLEXIBILITY AND COMFORT

1. Keep your knapsack as light as possible and carry it on both shoulders.

2. Perform a daily shower stretch routine to prepare the muscles for work.

3. Perform a cool-down routine once work is over to reduce stiffness/pain—i.e., when you arrive at school/home.

4. Perform exercises specifically to strengthen muscles that are over-worked.

5. Develop proper eating habits that include appropriate calcium and magnesium (see Chapter 4).

6. Buy a second used set of text books for home to limit carrying books to and from school.

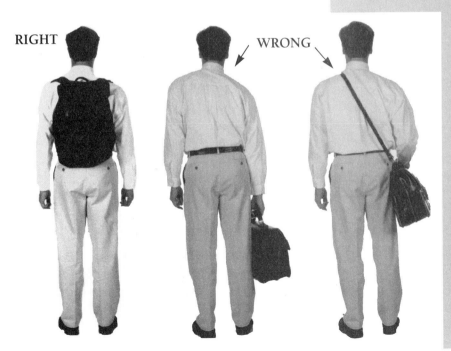

RIGHT

WRONG

17

ADULTS

Most adults have responsibilities to their career, family, and finances. They always seem to be in a rush. They are too busy to take a holiday, eat breakfast, sleep, stretch, exercise, and so on. Not surprisingly, many people suffer from a stiff neck that they have had since high school, or have frequent headaches. Without breakfast, they are prone to early fatigue in the muscle tissues. If these people work on computers or other stationary work occupations (70% of the population), they are particularly subject to the effects of static muscle loading (see p. 10), which can often lead to joint inflammation, tendon sheath inflammation, arthritis, disc trouble, an increased heart rate, higher blood pressure, and psychological disorders.

HOW TO IMPROVE ADULT COMFORT AND FLEXIBILITY

1. Eat balanced meals that contain adequate calcium and magnesium. Also have regular snacks between meals to maintain normal blood sugar levels and muscular fuel levels.

2. Perform the shower stretch routine in the morning as part of a warm-up and in the evening as a way to relax.

3. Stretch or move every 1–2 hours at work to reduce muscle stiffness.

4. Exercise regularly.

5. Consult a chiropractor for aches and pains that persist.

SENIORS

At age 65, many people feel that they can retire and do the things they have always wanted to do. However, many may soon realize that they cannot do the things that they once took for granted (i.e., ride a bicycle, play tennis, etc.), particularly if they did not take care of their musculoskeletal system in their younger years. Major health problems can evolve from minor problems. In extreme cases, this can lead to feelings of frustration and depression. However, it is seldom too late to begin rebuilding your body.

Case Study

M.B., an 80-year-old woman, suffered from cancer, a number of small strokes, and arthritis. After being given some simple stretches, she was almost immediately able to walk more easily about her cottage. After 2 weeks of daily stretching, she was able to walk to the end of her driveway—something that she had not been able to do for many years. She died 2 years later, but she felt much better during her last 2 years because she was more functional.

Stretching is a safe, effective, and important way for elderly people to stimulate muscles that have shortened and stiffened with age. A 65- or 85-year-old muscle can still be trained to work better, even if it has not been taken care of up to this point. Evidence suggests that stretching also improves an elderly person's psychological disposition, which can improve the quality of life.

HOW TO IMPROVE SENIORS' FLEXIBILITY AND COMFORT

1. Perform a morning stretch routine to improve balance and muscle tone.

2. Engage in exercise and physical activity to strengthen bones as well as muscles.

3. Eat a proper diet that includes sufficient calcium, magnesium, and protein.

Stretch Break

Stand close to a chair so that the spine is straight.

Hold the left foot with the left hand.

Pull gently.

Hold for 30 seconds (three to five deep breaths).

Breathe normally; repeat with the other leg.

Many retirement homes now include daily stretching and coordination activities to promote muscle tone and reduce the rate of degeneration or aging. In fact, a 1989 study of women between the ages of 69 and 95 who undertook a workout program showed that their forearm bones actually became measurably denser. If your retirement or nursing home does not offer a flexibility/exercise program, you shoulder suggest that they set up a stretching class as soon as possible.

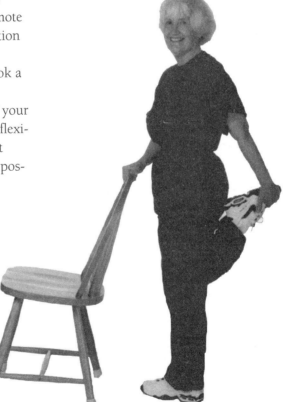

Calcium & Magnesium: Muscle Fibers & Stretching

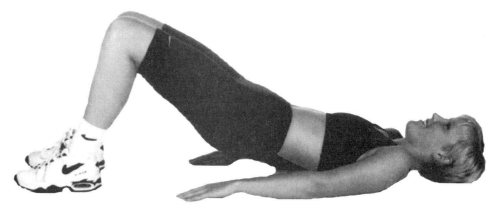

Diet plays an integral role in developing and maintaining bones and muscles. Since most people have sedentary lives—sitting at home or work, commuting, and sleeping—many of them suffer from stiff and sore muscles. Many, however, would not be as susceptible to these muscular aches and pains if, along with stretching, they consumed appropriate amounts of calcium and magnesium to help muscles stretch and relax.

CALCIUM

Calcium not only helps develop and strengthen teeth and bones (99% of calcium in the body), it also plays a vital role in the normal rhythmic and smooth contraction of muscles in the human body (1% of total body calcium). Calcium helps the infrastructure of the muscle fibers, known as cross-bridges, to work optimally. These cross-bridges link two muscle fibers together and create a shortening, or contraction, in the muscle.

They lock the muscle fibers in place so that "slippage" does not occur until the activity is over. Insufficient calcium in the blood reduces the number of bridges formed, which reduces the strength of the muscle contraction.

In addition, calcium helps the nerves and muscles communicate. A shortage of calcium causes the nerves to become irritated, which leads to muscle tension, stiffness, and eventual pain.

DAILY DIETARY CALCIUM REQUIREMENTS

Infants	
0–6 months	360 mg
6–12 months	540 mg
Children (ages 1–10)	800 mg
Adolescents (ages 11–17)	1200 mg

Adults	800 mg
Seniors (age 65+)	1200 mg
Post-menopausal women	1200–1500 mg
Pregnant/lactating women	1200–1500 mg

Even though you accumulate most of your bone mass by age 18, you still acquire extra amounts of calcium between ages 18 and 30. Current research suggests that an increase in bone mass can still occur even after menopause.

FOOD SOURCES HIGH IN CALCIUM

1 cup of milk (2% or skim)	297–302 mg
1 cup of yogurt	274 mg
1 ounce of cheese	204 mg
1 cup of broccoli	42 mg
12 medium-size raw oysters	226 mg
½ cup of almonds	166 mg

NOTE: *If you are lactose intolerant (cannot digest milk or milk products), then take calcium citrate or carbonate supplements to meet your daily calcium dietary needs.*

NOTE: *Dairy products and antibiotics do not mix. Dairy products can hinder the absorption of many antibiotics, medications, and other vitamins/minerals. For example, tetracycline binds with calcium and loses it effectiveness.*

Facts

1. Only 20–30% of your dietary calcium is absorbed through the food you eat. This is all the more reason to include calcium-rich foods in your diet.
2. As you get older, your calcium requirement increases because the rate of absorption decreases.

3. Vitamin D, vitamin C, and magnesium promote calcium absorption.
4. Calcium does not cause:
  a. hardening of the arteries;
  b. deposits in the muscles (except in rare cases, such as parathyroid gland disease, in which the body's calcium balance is affected);
  c. kidney stones (it may actually reduce the risk of them).

Functions of Calcium in the Human Body

☞ Forms teeth

☞ Develops bones

☞ Reduces cramps in muscles

☞ Assists in nerve conductivity and helps stretching

☞ Assists in blood clotting and healing of soft tissues

☞ Assists in the rhythmic contraction of muscles

MAGNESIUM

Magnesium is required to release the cross-bridges between the muscle fibers at the end of a muscle contraction so that the muscle can relax. Approximately 70% of the body's magnesium is located in the bones, while 30% is found in soft tissues and associated structures. If the body is deficient in magnesium, the muscles will not relax enough. Instead, they will tend to stay in a contracted, tight, or stiff condition. Over time, this stiffness can be felt as knots, ropes, or even cramps. Magnesium deficiency is also closely related to heart disease.

DAILY DIETARY MAGNESIUM REQUIREMENTS

Infants	200–400 mg
Children (ages 1–10)	200–400 mg
Adolescents (ages 11–17)	200–400 mg
Adult males	350–400 mg
Adult females	300–350 mg
Seniors (age 65+)	450 mg
Post-menopausal women	450 mg
Pregnant/lactating women	450 mg

NOTE: *Your magnesium intake should be half the amount of your calcium intake.*

FOOD SOURCES HIGH IN MAGNESIUM

1 cup of fresh green vegetables (e.g., broccoli)	22 mg
1 cup of milk	28–33 mg
1 pound of shrimp	190 mg
1 pound of oyster	140 mg
1 cup of almonds	386 mg

Stretch Break

Keep arms at shoulder level, elbows bent at 90°, and palms facing down.

Twist torso and neck to the left while keeping pelvis straight.

Hold for 30 seconds (three to five deep breaths).

Breathe normally; twist to the other side.

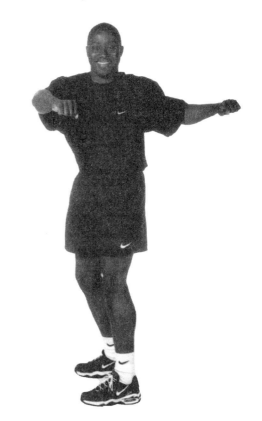

Understanding Your Body & Its Limits

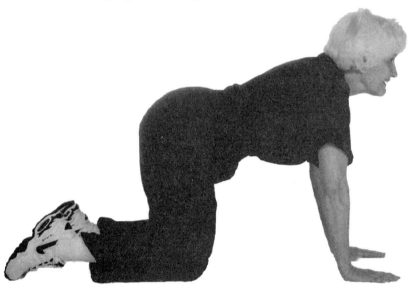

*B*efore we get to the basic stretches for each part of our body, we need to discuss each person's body and its own uniqueness. Before stretching or doing any type of physical activity, everyone should know their individual physical limitations and learn how to listen to their body.

FINDING YOUR INHERENT BLUEPRINT

Besides your annual physical examination with your physician, you should be examined by a chiropractor to determine any potential problems that may lead to debilitating injuries. The chiropractor can make an accurate assessment and diagnosis of your spine, joints, and muscles to determine your specific, inherent blueprint (or

body mechanics composition). This way, you will know your body's structural composition and capacity in order to function efficiently in your environment.

Your chiropractor can correlate the specifics of an individual joint or nerve problem and help you understand which muscles are weak. For instance, if a muscle is short, adjacent muscles or muscle groups will make compensatory changes. This, in turn, causes other tissue changes throughout the body that could result in bone or joint misalignment, which leads to nerve irritation or inflammation.

Your body has the natural ability to heal itself if the proper conditions are established, such as correcting the joint alignment and movement pattern so that you allow the corresponding nerve to function better. In order to perform anything at an optimal level, all joint and nerve problems must be corrected. Once you understand your inherent blueprint, you can work with it and use appropriate stretches to maintain optimal functionality and health.

UNDERSTANDING AND ALLEVIATING PAIN

Mechanical problems, such as low back pain, sciatica, a stiff neck, scoliosis, headaches, tennis elbow, and bursitis, afflict many people and can significantly alter their ability to function. Some people may ignore their pain, thinking that it will go away, when, in fact, pain is an alarm that something *is wrong*.

Nerve, joint, and muscle irritation/inflammation will cause you to feel any or all of the following symptoms:

☞ Dull pain	☞ Muscle knots
☞ Numbness	☞ Spasms
☞ Stiffness	☞ Sharp pain
☞ Tingling	☞ Cramping
☞ Tightness	☞ Shooting pain
☞ Burning	☞ Weakness

Stretching can help diminish muscle spasms, pain, and other symptoms. You can also try applying an ice pack or heating pad to the irritated area before you begin stretching. Both hot and cold treatments work up to an inch into the muscle. Whichever treatment you use, if you do not see an improvement after 1–2 weeks, consult your physician (also see Chapter 11 for specific areas of injuries and pain).

Cold and Heat Therapy

Always choose the hottest or coldest temperature that you can tolerate. The following are general rules regarding when you should use heat or cold for an irritated area:

1. If you have a dull or sharp pain in a localized area, apply ice to it in 10-minute intervals. For example, ice an area for 10 minutes, and then remove it for at least 10 minutes. Repeat this three to five times.

CAUTION:

If you exceed 12–15 minutes of icing on a specific area, the body's natural reaction will be to increase circulation (dilate the blood vessel) in order to protect the tissue from cell damage. The increased flow to the already inflamed area will make it even more inflamed and, hence, it will counteract the initial benefits of cold by causing more pain.

---

2. For muscle stiffness, use a heating pad or, better yet, take a warm shower (see Chapter 8).

3. You can apply both heat and cold to a traumatized area. Simply alternate cold with heat for a couple of days if the area is not responding to either alone. This can also be done once the pain of an acute injury has been reduced. The concept behind contrast is simple. The ice constricts the blood flow and reduces swelling while the heat promotes blood flow. If you alternate between the two, you will help accelerate the removal of pain-producing waste products in the injured region. Always begin and finish with cold. The two standard methods of hot and cold applications are:

a. 5 minutes of moderately cold and then 5 minutes of moderately hot temperatures.

b. 20–30 seconds of very cold and hot temperatures. Do not make the hot temperature over 105°F (40°C).

WARNING:

Hot or cold should never be applied to areas where there is reduced sensation. This may make you apply a harmful amount of hot/cold without realizing the damage being done. Neither should also be applied where there is a chance of an infection or malignancy. Cold is not recommended for people with peripheral vascular diseases, such as sickle-cell anemia or Raynaud's disease.

Exercising and Pain

At times, especially during exercising, the feeling of pain may seem to lessen. But it is only a temporary condition that is caused by: 1. endorphins; 2. nerve activation in the body.

1. Endorphin Theory

Endorphins and enkephalins are chemicals that are made in the human body. They are opiates that inhibit pain when released. For example, endorphins are responsible for the "high" joggers feel when running. Endorphins and enkephalins can be stimulated both physically and mentally. For instance, if you get excited in anticipation of a sports event (pre-game "jitters"), this chemical can be triggered to reduce your overall ability to feel pain.

But just because the pain is gone does not mean that the problem is gone and that, therefore, it is safe to exercise. Endorphins only *mask* the pain. They do not fix the underlying mechanical problem.

2. The "Gate" Theory of Pain

To understand this theory, think of a nerve acting as a "gateway" through which information can pass from a joint or muscle to the brain and back again. According to this theory, the body's joints have two main types of nerves. One type senses and reports the movement of the joint to the brain. The other is a smaller, pain-sensing nerve. There are more movement-nerve receptors than pain-nerve receptors in a joint.

The "gate" to the brain overrides pain messages if the primary motion-detecting nerve keeps feeding signals into it. An example of this happens when you exercise while in pain. The pain information to the brain is overridden, and you do not notice the pain while you are moving. Stop the activity and the pain returns, because the primary movement information to the brain is reduced, allowing the pain signals to dominate once again.

Many people feel exercise helps their pain problems because it feels better when they exercise. WRONG! Exercise done at the right time, and correctly, can strengthen and stabilize your entire musculoskeletal system as well as enhance overall health to prevent the recurrence of pain and mechanical problems. However, exercising an area when it hurts does more damage than good in the long run.

Six Rules to Stretching

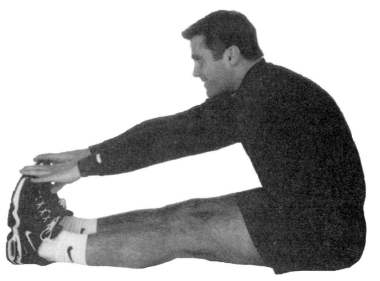

*A*lways keep these six rules in mind when you are performing *any* kind of stretch.

1. WARM-UP

Before you stretch, your muscles should be warm. An efficient warm-up can include marching, walking in place while swinging your arms, taking a warm shower, or mimicking the sport you are about to do (e.g., for squash: swing the racquet, twist the torso, and lunge). The warm-up increases the muscle temperature, which increases blood flow to the tissue. The muscle fibers can then respond more quickly and efficiently to the stretch.

From a practical perspective, the shower stretch routine is the best time to do your stretches (see Chapter 8). It is easy to remember, becomes part of a habit, and therefore is something that you can see immediate results from.

2. BE GENTLE

Do not force a muscle to stretch. All you should feel is a gentle pull in the muscle. It should take approximately 6–10 seconds for the internal muscle-protective mechanism to adapt to the new position. Then the nervous system will allow the muscle fibers to relax and change their length. In the next 20–24 seconds, you should notice a gradual decrease in the pulling sensation. At the end of 30 seconds, you should feel almost no pulling sensation. If you still feel something, you are stretching too far, which can result in a sore and stiff muscle. Simply ease back to the point or position where you feel virtually nothing in order to allow the muscle to adapt to its new length. The "no pain, no gain" theory does not apply to stretching.

3. HOLD FOR 30 SECONDS

Current research shows that a stretch must be held for at least 30 seconds. If you cannot hold the stretch comfortably for this long, then ease back. Anything less than 30 seconds will not give the nerves enough time to adapt to the new length and alter the muscle tone. Only one repetition per muscle is required when done daily. However, if you notice that a muscle on one side is tighter than the same muscle on the other side, you may want to stretch it two to four times to fully relax it. Ultimately, you want symmetry.

4. BREATHE

Deep, rhythmic, abdominal breathing helps to improve circulation to muscle tissues. This enhances nutrient flow (especially calcium and magnesium, see Chapter 4) to muscle fibers. Breathing also is meditative and helps you relax. Holding your breath will make the stretch ineffective.

5. DO NOT BOUNCE

Bouncing, or ballistic stretching, stresses the joints, ligaments, and muscles. It also triggers the protective stretch mechanism within the muscle to reflexively contract. As a result, the muscles cannot relax or stretch. Always stretch slowly and gently.

6. STRETCH BOTH SIDES

Always stretch the right and left sides (or the front and back) of an area to maintain balance and symmetry. This will enhance flexibility and performance while reducing the risk of injury. Pay attention to your muscles. If the muscle you stretch responds quickly, you can assume it is healthy and does not require much work. If it is stiff and does not move easily, you may need to repeat the stretch until it relaxes. Learn to "listen" to the muscle's response to the stretch so that you will learn more about your inherent blueprint (see Chapter 5).

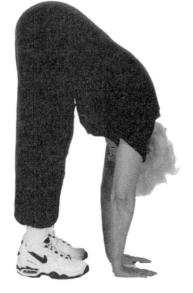

The Basic Stretches & Their Anatomy

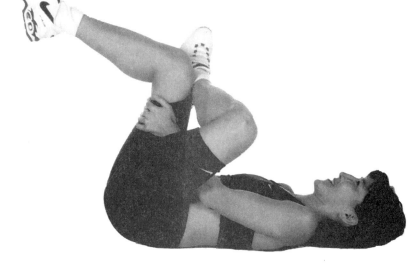

Now that we have covered the fundamentals of stretching, let's move on to the practical part of the book. This chapter includes pictures for stretching every area and muscle group in the human body. It also includes illustrations of the corresponding muscle you are stretching so that you will know what the muscle looks like or how the muscle fibers travel. This way, you can fully appreciate and visualize the underlying muscle being worked on to help you better relax and stretch that muscle.

The stretches and anatomical illustrations are placed in the order from your head to feet. All the stretches here are both safe and effective. They can easily be referenced for a simple review of any specific stretch you require. Ideally, the stretch should be one that you like and are comfortable doing. For example, if sitting on the floor is a problem, you can use an alternate move, since most stretches are provided with standing, sitting, and lying options. Remember always to apply the Six Rules to Stretching (see Chapter 6).

Now is when you begin to manage yourself by evaluating and working with your relative strengths and weaknesses. For instance, you may notice that one side of your body is not as flexible as the other. You should then repeat the stretch on the stiffer side one or two more times to balance out flexibility on both sides. By doing this, you will notice outstanding results in a very short time.

Jaw

Muscles

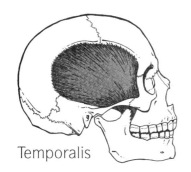

Temporalis

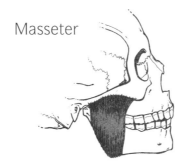

Masseter

Stretches

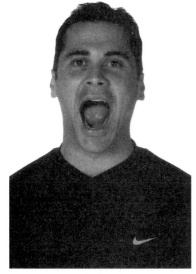

Open Mouth Stretch

Stand in a comfortable position. Open your jaw to its limit without straining. Hold for 30 seconds. Breathe deeply. If you are prone to lockjaw or TMJ syndrome, do not push this stretch too hard.

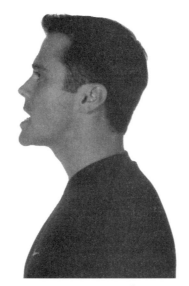

Jaw Protrusion Stretch

Stand in a comfortable position. Hold your head up and stick your lower jaw comfortably forward. Hold for 30 seconds. Breathe deeply.

Case Study #1: Tooth and Head Pain

History: S.M., a 42-year-old accountant, experienced intense pain in his tooth and on the side of his head. He went to an endodontist (mouth specialist) who examined his teeth and found nothing wrong. The examination cost $700. He then went to an ear, nose, and throat specialist who, after finding nothing wrong, referred him to a chiropractor.

Diagnosis: Pressure along the second and third cervical bones, spinal dysfunction, and referred pain to the teeth from the neck.

Treatment: Neck adjustment and stretching.

Result: Immediate reduction of tooth and head pain.

Note: The patient continued to manage his neck bone abnormality with stretching and chiropractic check-ups. After 7 years, he has had no reoccurrence. The cost of his chiropractic exam, X-rays , and treatment was $82.

Neck

The neck region is often overlooked when stretching, but these muscles are crucial in supporting the head and maintaining balance of the human frame. You should start all flexibility programs with neck and jaw stretches. Never roll your head, because, first and most importantly, the bones will grind. Secondly, the nerves, tendons, ligaments, and blood vessels become irritated. Once this happens, pain and lack of movement will follow. Neck injuries of this type are particularly painful, because of the proximity of this region to the spinal nerves, spinal cord, and brain. Third, the muscles do not lengthen and relax when this type of neck rolling is done. Fourth, you may compress a nerve or cause it to function improperly, especially when the head is placed into extreme extension. Finally, the arteries in the head can be impinged by head rolling. This can temporarily cut off blood supply to the brain, leading to dizziness and even vertigo in chronic cases.

The chin-to-chest stretch has been deliberately omitted from our set of neck stretches, because the majority of people inadvertently stretch these muscle throughout their daily activity. S]itting at a desk or in front of a computer, or even reading in bed, lengthens the back neck muscles. Therefore, these muscles rarely require stretching. A painter would be someone who may benefit from the chin-to-chest stretch, since the job requires a great deal of looking up.

Muscles

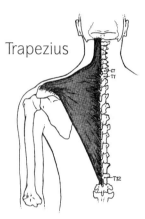

Trapezius

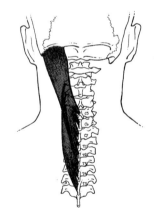

Splenius capitis (top muscle) and cervicis (lower muscle)

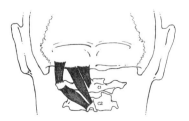

Suboccipitalis

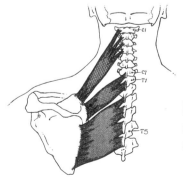

Levator scapulae (top muscle) and Rhomboids (lower two muscles)

Back of the Neck Stretches

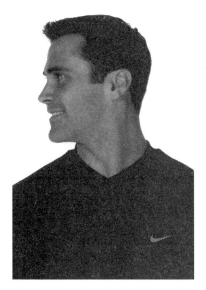

Neck Turn

Stand comfortably. Keeping your chin and jaw parallel to the ground, look over your right shoulder so that your face is 90° from your torso midline. Hold for 30 seconds. Breathe deeply. Repeat on the other side. This stretch can make checking lanes when driving much easier.

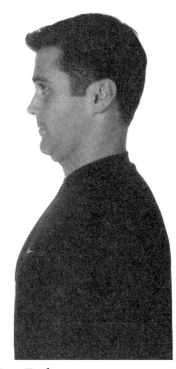

Jaw Tuck

Stand comfortably. While holding the head straight up, retract the jaw so that it tilts the face slightly forward. Hold for 30 seconds. Breathe deeply. This will stretch the muscles under the skull at the back of the neck.

Case Study #2: Classic Migraine Headache

History: S.T., a 22-year-old sound designer/editor, had a lifelong history of headaches that occurred at least two times a week. The headaches were triggered by low blood-sugar levels, chocolate, nuts, and red wine.

Diagnosis: Pressure on the nerves of the upper neck caused the muscle tension headaches and migraines. Sensitivity to certain foods.

Treatment: Neck and upper back adjustments, stretching, and dietary changes.

Result: No pain for 2 years.

Note: S.T. has learned how to manage his condition with stretching.

Side of the Neck

Muscles

Levator scapulae and Rhomboids See page 30.

Trapezius See page 30.

Stretches

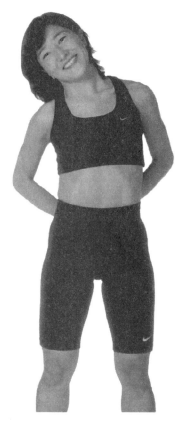

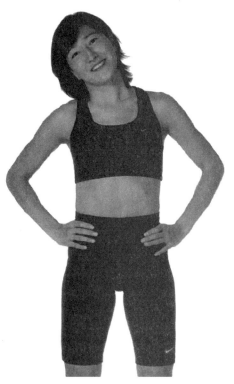

Neck Tilt

Stand comfortably. Lean the right ear toward the right shoulder. Keep the nose pointing straight ahead. Do not force the stretch or point the nose to the shoulder. Hold for 30 seconds. Breathe deeply. Repeat on the other side.

Neck Tilt with Arms Held

Follow the same method as the neck tilt stretch, except use the hand of the side that you are leaning your head towards to grasp the other wrist firmly. Pull the wrist/arm down until the upper arm touches the side of the body. Hold comfortably for 30 seconds. Breathe deeply. Repeat on the other side.

This stretch works the top of the shoulder and the upper arm (i.e., deltoid).

Front of the Neck

Muscles

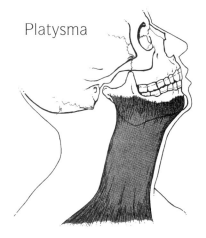

Platysma

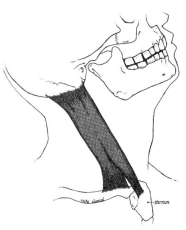

Sternocleidomastoid

Front of Neck Muscles Continued

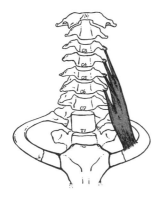
Scalene anterior

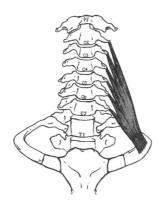
Scalene medius

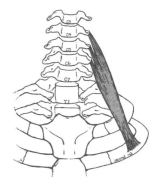
Scalene posterior

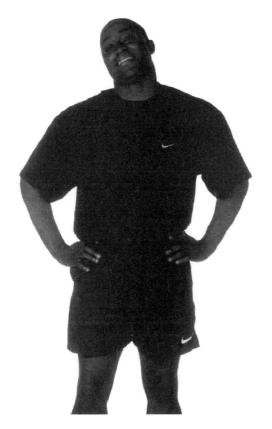

Stretch

Neck Tilt with Slight Extension

Stand comfortably. Tilt the right ear to the right shoulder and turn the face to the left or upwards about half an inch. Slightly extend the neck backwards about half an inch. Hold comfortably for 30 seconds. Breathe deeply. This will stretch the front left side of the neck. Repeat on the other side. This stretch helps your posture. If you feel a pinch in the neck or experience dizziness consult your chiropractor immediately. Never lean the head straight back into extreme extension!

This muscle is commonly overlooked or forgotten. Yet, when stretched properly, it can provide substantial relief of neck pain.

Shoulder

Top of the Shoulder
Muscles

Levator scapulae and Rhomboids See page 30.

Trapezius See page 30.

Deltoid

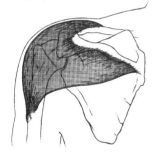

Rotator cuff (four parts)

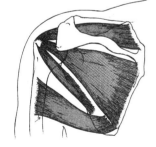

- Supraspinatus
- Infraspinatus
- Teres major and minor

Stretches

Neck Tilt with Arms Held
See page 32.

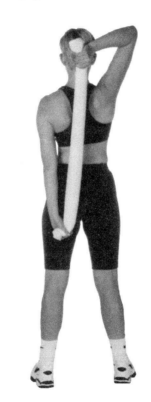

Towel Assisted Stretch

Stand comfortably. Hold a towel as shown in the photo. Use your right hand to pull up on the towel. This stretches the top of the left shoulder. The left arm can be straight; however, it is most effective with the left elbow bent above 90°.

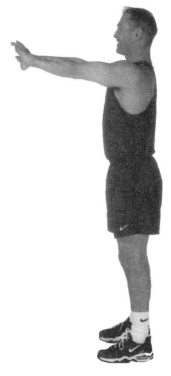

Front Press Out

Sit up straight in a chair or stand with feet shoulder-width apart. Clasp your fingers and push the palms away from your body. Once the elbows are straight, you will feel a stretch to the top and back of the shoulders. Hold comfortably for 30 seconds. Breathe deeply.

Back of the Shoulder

Muscles

Levator scapulae and Rhomboids See page 30.

Trapezius See page 30.

Deltoid See page 34.

Rotator cuff See page 34.

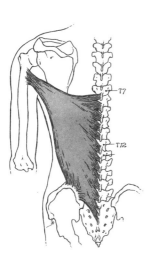

Latissimus dorsi

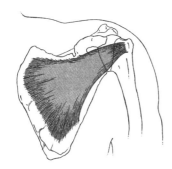

Subscapularis

Stretches

Front Press Out
See page 34.

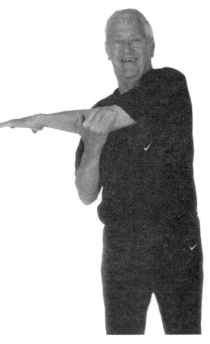

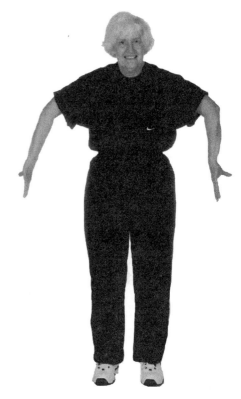

Deltoid Stretch
Stand comfortably with feet shoulder-width apart. Keeping the left arm straight, reach it across the body. Use the right hand to pull the elbow into the chest while your face and shoulders are looking straight ahead. Hold comfortably for 30 seconds. Breathe deeply. Repeat to the other side. For a deeper stretch, bend the left arm at the elbow, twist the torso to the right, and turn the face to the right. This stretches the back of the left shoulder rotator cuff muscles. Repeat to the other side. Always do this stretch first in any shoulder flexibility program.

Internal Rotation Stretch

Stand with feet shoulder-width apart, knees slightly bent, and shoulders back. Hold both arms straight with palms facing in. Turn the palms inward to stretch the muscles that rotate the shoulders backward. Hold comfortably for 30 seconds. Breathe deeply.

Back of Shoulder Stretches Continued

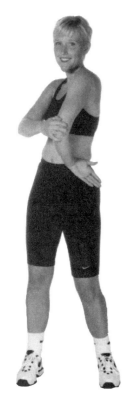

Rotator Cuff Stretch

Stand comfortably with feet shoulder-width apart. Bend the left arm at the elbow and place the top of the wrist (back of hand) at your side above the waist. Use the right hand to hold the left elbow and bring it forward. When you become more flexible, the left elbow should almost point in front of you. For a greater stretch, twist the torso to the right. Hold comfortably for 30 seconds. Breathe deeply. Repeat on the other side.

Bottom of the Shoulder

Muscles

Latissimus dorsi See page 35.

Rotator cuff See page 34.

Subscapularis See page 35.

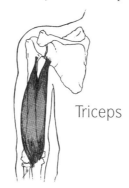

Triceps

Stretches

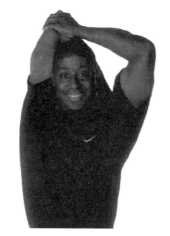

Arm Over Head Stretch

Stand comfortably with feet shoulder-width apart. Keeping the back and neck straight, gently pull the right elbow over the head as shown in the photo. Do not force the head forward, in order to reduce neck strain. For a greater stretch, lean the torso to the left. Hold comfortably for 30 seconds. Breathe deeply. Repeat to the other side.

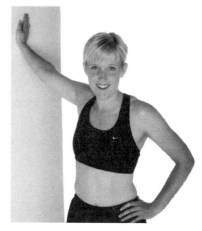

Lower Chest Stretch

Stand at arm's length from a doorway or wall. Stretch your arm out against the support until it is at a 45° angle above the shoulder or horizontal plane. Keep the palm flat against the support and the arm straight to stretch the bicep at the elbow, which indirectly helps the movement of the front of the shoulder. When you begin, you may find that your torso and face are towards the wall. As flexibility increases, your torso will be able to point away from the wall as in the photo.

*Bottom of Shoulder Stretches
Continued*

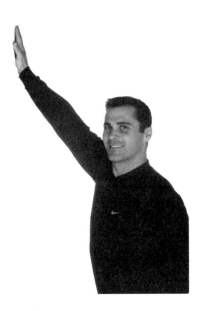

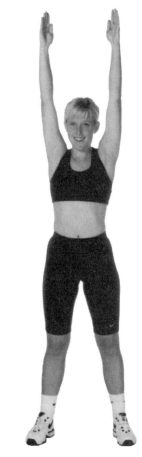

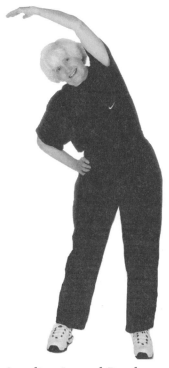

Reach Stretch

Stand facing a wall with arm straight at shoulder height and fingers outstretched so that the fingertips touch the wall. Let your finger slowly walk up the wall; you may have to move closer to the wall as your fingers climb higher. Go as high as comfortably possible. Stop. Hold for 30 seconds. Breathe deeply. Mark this level off with a pencil so that you can monitor your progress. Repeat to the other side.

This stretch is also called the "wall walk."

Tall Stretch

Stand comfortably with feet shoulder-width apart or until you feel balanced. Point toes slightly out. Raise hands over the head with palms inward and arms shoulder-width apart. Stretch comfortably upward, standing up on your toes if possible. Hold for 30 seconds. Breathe deeply. You can do this stretch lying down on the bed or floor with toes pointed. If you are prone to calf cramps, don't point your toes.

Standing Lateral Bend

Keep both hands hanging to the side. Keep the feet at least a shoulder-width apart for balance. Reach one hand over the head. The overhead arm should always remain in the plane of the body. Do not rotate the torso forward. The palm of the overhead hand must always face the floor to reduces the stress on the shoulder joint. The other hand can rest on the hip or side of knee for support, if needed. Hold for 30 seconds. Breathe deeply. Repeat on the other side.

Bottom of Shoulder Stretches Continued

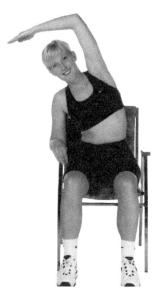

Sitting Lateral Bend

Sit with your buttocks against the back of a chair and your feet flat on the floor. Make sure that the spine remains in the vertical plane when bending laterally in order to maximize this stretch. Bring the left arm over the head as you tilt the shoulder and ear to the right side so that the body is parallel to the floor. Use the right hand to hold the arm of the chair for stability. Do not twist the body. Make sure the shoulder on the left side is not pointing to the floor. Otherwise, you are rotating. Hold for 30 seconds. Breathe deeply. Repeat to the other side.

This is a good stretch to do at the office or if you have low back pain.

Front of the Shoulder

Muscles

Deltoid See page 34.

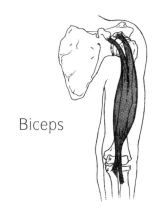

Biceps

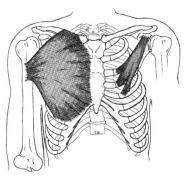

Pectoralis major/minor

Stretches

Lower Chest Stretch
See page 36.

Shoulder Blade Squeeze
See page 40.

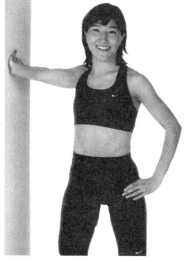

Middle Chest Stretch

Stand at arm's length from a doorway or wall. Stretch your arm out against the support until it is parallel to the floor. Keep the palm flat against the support, elbow straight, and fingers pointing backwards. The closer the body is to the support and the more you twist your torso away from it, the greater the stretch will be on the chest. Hold comfortably for 30 seconds. Breathe deeply. Repeat to the other side.

Front of Shoulder Stretches Continued

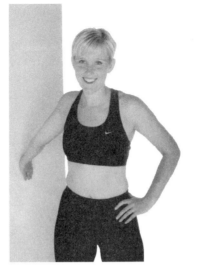

Upper Chest Stretch

Stand at arm's length from a doorway or wall. Stretch your arm out against the support until it is at a 45° angle below the horizontal plane. Keep the palm flat against the support, fingers pointed downward, and elbows straight. The closer the body is to the support and the more you twist your torso away from it, the greater the stretch will be on the chest. Hold comfortably for 30 seconds. Breathe deeply. Repeat to the other side.

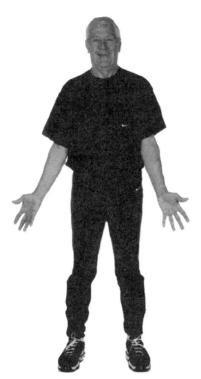

External Rotation Stretch

Stand comfortably with feet shoulder-width apart, knees slightly bent, and shoulders back. Hold the arms straight with palms facing inward. Then turn the elbows outward to stretch the muscles that rotate the shoulder forward and inward. Hold comfortably for 30 seconds. Breathe deeply.

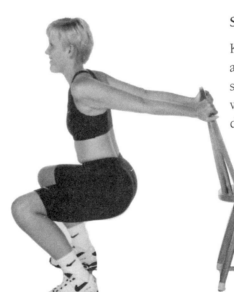

Squatting Chest Stretch

Keep the feet shoulder-width apart with the toes pointing straight ahead or slightly outward. Place both hands on a desk, table top, or chair. Keep elbows straight and palms down or inward—not outward. Slowly squat down to a comfortable level. Make sure that your stance is solid so that you do not slip and strain your shoulders. Hold for 30 seconds. Breathe deeply. The deeper the squat, the greater the stretch on the chest.

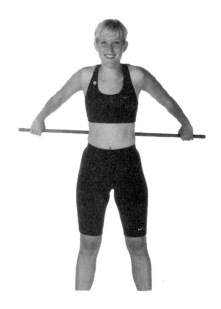

Front of Shoulder Stretches Continued

Bar Chest Stretch

Stand comfortably with feet shoulder-width apart. Hold the bar in one hand and reach around behind the back with the other hand to grasp the free end of the bar. Hold the bar behind at a comfortable height. Keep both palms facing backwards. It is important not to lower the bar behind the head while holding both its ends, or else it will put unnecessary strain on the shoulders. Hold comfortably for 30 seconds. Breathe deeply. Where you hold the bar will determine which part of your chest you are stretching. Holding the bar above shoulder height stretches the lower chest (although it is not recommended), at shoulder height stretches the mid-chest (most difficult), and below shoulder height stretches the upper chest.

The Chest

Muscles

Pectoralis major/minor
See page 38.

Stretches

External Rotation Stretch
See page 39.

Lower Chest Stretch
See page 36.

Middle Chest Stretch
See page 38.

Upper Chest Stretch
See page 39.

Bar Chest Stretch
See page 40.

Squatting Chest Stretch
See page 39.

Shoulder Blade Squeeze

Stand comfortably with feet shoulder-width apart. Place your hands behind your back and join the fingers together. If your hands are below the waist, you will stretch the mid- and upper chest. If your hands are above the horizontal plane, you will stretch the lower chest. Squeeze the shoulder blades together and hold comfortably for 30 seconds. Breathe deeply.

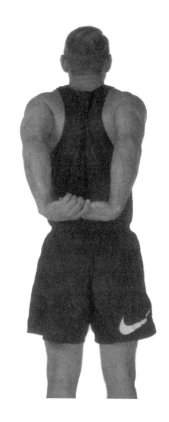

Case Study #3: Chest Numbness

History: K.P., a 42-year-old nurse and homemaker, suffered numbness in the left chest for many years. Her father also suffered the same symptoms. She consulted a gynecologist, cardiologist, medical doctor, and neurologist. She consulted a chiropractor 6 years ago.

Diagnosis: The left third and fourth ribs irritated the spine and its nerves, which caused the tingling sensation from the spine to her left chest wall.

Treatment: Rib adjustments and stretches for the upper body.

Result: Her symptoms disappeared shortly after treatment began and have not returned in the last 6 years.

The Arm

The Upper Arm

Muscles

Biceps See page 38.

Triceps See page 36.

Stretches

Arm Over Head Stretch
See page 36.

Middle Chest Stretch
See page 38.

External Rotation Stretch
See page 39.

Towel Assisted Stretch
See page 34.

The Middle Arm (or Elbow)

Muscles

Biceps See page 39.

Triceps See page 36.

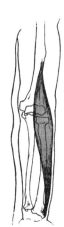
Brachioradialis

Stretches

Arm Over Head Stretch
See page 36.

Lower Chest Stretch
See page 36.

Middle Chest Stretch
See page 38.

Upper Chest Stretch
See page 39.

Bar Chest Stretch
See page 40.

External Rotation Stretch
See page 39.

Squatting Chest Stretch
See page 39.

The Lower Arm (Forearm)

Muscles

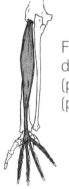

Flexor digitorum (profundus) (palm surface)

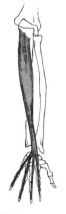

Extensor digitorum

Stretches

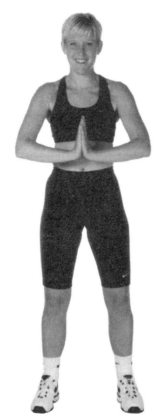

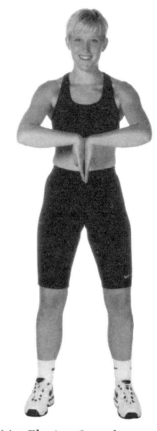

Wrist Extension Stretch

Stand comfortably with feet shoulder-width apart. Put the hands together in a prayer position and press the wrist downward until the forearms form a 90° angle with the hands. This may not be possible to do at first, but as flexibility increases, you will be push further down. Hold comfortably for 30 seconds. Breathe deeply.

This stretch is excellent for computer workers or typists.

Wrist Flexion Stretch

Stand comfortably with feet shoulder-width apart. Place the backs of your hands together at the level of the stomach and press. Press the forearms downward, if possible. Slowly raise hands up to a comfortable level. Hold for 30 seconds. Breathe deeply. This stretch move is also known as a "reverse prayer" stretch.

Forearm Stretches Continued

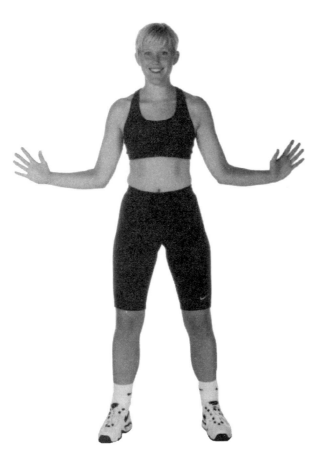

Top of Wrist Stretch

Stand comfortably with feet shoulder-width apart. Keeping forearms parallel to the floor, tilt the wrist 20–30° inwards toward the body. Try to point the fingers to the floor. Hold comfortably for 30 seconds. Breathe deeply. This stretch is for the outside forearm.

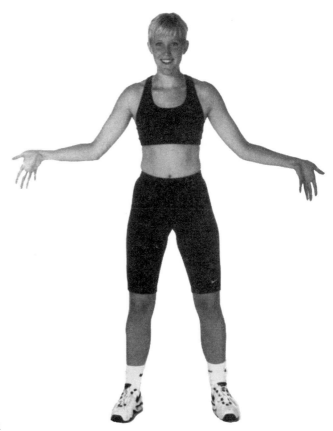

Bottom of Wrist Stretch

Stand with feet shoulder-width apart. Keeping forearms parallel to the floor, tilt the wrists 10–15° up toward the elbows. With the hands out, point the thumbs up. Hold comfortably for 30 seconds. Breathe deeply. This is a good stretch for the inside of the forearm.

Forearm Stretches Continued

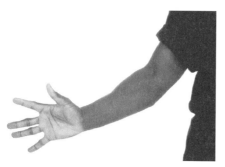

Open Hand Stretch

While standing or sitting comfortably, spread the fingers as wide as possible. Imagine that you are trying to grasp a basketball that is too big for your hand. Hold for 30 seconds. Breathe deeply. Repeat with the other hand. This stretches the palms and fingers.

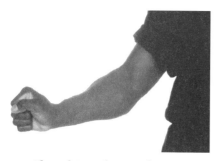

Closed Hand Stretch

While standing or sitting comfortably, make a tight fist by clenching your hand. Hold for 30 seconds. Breathe deeply. If your hand begins to cramp, you are squeezing too tightly. Repeat with the other hand. This stretches the back of the hand.

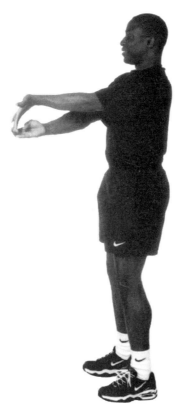

Wrist Extension Stretch

Stand comfortably with feet shoulder-width apart. Hold fingertips of the left hand with the right hand. The fingertips can be pointing up or down. Press the palm of the left hand forward and straighten the elbow. Hold comfortably for 30 seconds. Breathe deeply. Repeat on the other side.

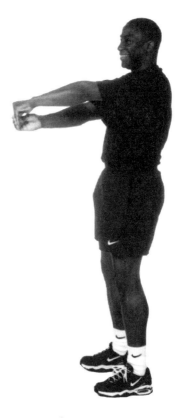

Wrist Flexion Stretch

Stand comfortably with feet shoulder-width apart. Bend the left palm down and secure the fingertips with the right hand. The fingertips can be pointing up or down. Press the left wrist forward and straighten the elbow. Hold for 30 seconds. Breathe deeply. Repeat on the other side. This is an excellent stretch for tennis elbow conditions.

Case Study #4: Arm and Hand Numbness

History: K.E., a 36-year-old professional singer, had numbness and tingling down the right arm into the thumb and first two fingers for a month. The problem was caused by lifting heavy production equipment.

Diagnosis: Multiple neck and shoulder strain at the fifth, sixth, and seventh joints of the neck. The pain was referred along the nerve root and down the right arm and hand.

Treatment: Neck adjustment, proper lifting technique instruction, and stretches.

Result: Complete normal function of the right arm and hand within 3 weeks. No recurrence of arm/hand pain in the last 17 months.

The Back

The Upper Back

Muscles

Levator scapulae and Rhomboids See page 30.

Stretches

Neck Tilt with Arms Held
See page 32.

Reach Stretch
See page 37.

Front Press Out
See page 34.

The Middle and Low Back

Muscles

Latissimus dorsi See page 35.

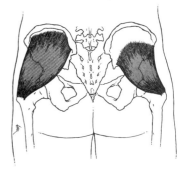

Gluteus medius/minimus

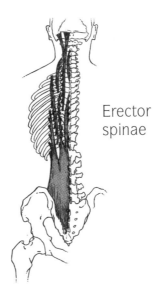

Erector spinae

Middle and Low Back Muscles Continued

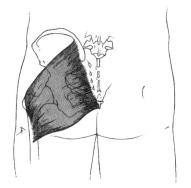

Gluteus maximus

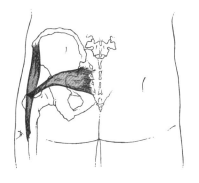

Piriformis/Tensor fasciae latae (TFL)

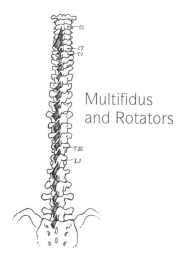

Multifidus and Rotators

Stretches

Tall Stretch
See page 37.

Standing Lateral Bend
See page 37.

Sitting Lateral Bend
See page 38.

Knee to Chest Stretch
Lie down on the floor or a firm surface (not on a soft bed, as it can strain the low back ligaments). Bring your left knee as close to your chest as possible.

Pull from above or below the left knee to help bring it closer. If you feel a pinch on the top of the hip, you are going too far. Hold comfortably for 30 seconds. Breathe deeply. Repeat on the right leg. This stretch can also be done standing up. It helps to open the base of the back and hip joint.

Figure Four Stretch

Lie flat on your back. Cross one foot over the other knee so that the ankle is resting on the lower thigh muscle. Wrap hands under the back leg and slowly pull

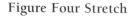

towards you. Breathe deeply. Hold comfortably for 30 to 60 seconds. Feel the stretch in the buttock muscle of the leg that is crossed over in front of you.

This gluteal muscle stretch (formerly called a "piriformis stretch") is a more advanced hip stretch and should be done after the knee to chest stretch.

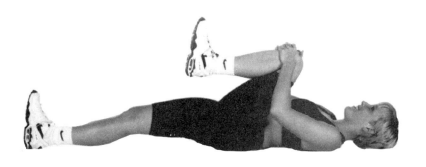

*Middle and Low Back Stretches
Continued*

However, it also places stress on the sciatic nerve. Therefore, stretch slowly and cautiously.

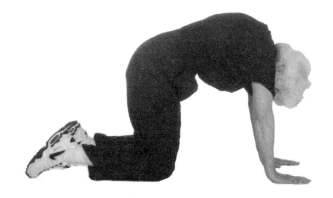

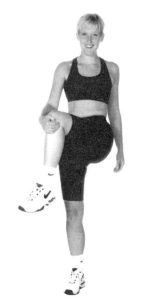

Knee to Opposite Chest Stretch

Stand up comfortably against a wall or lie down on a firm surface. Slowly bend the left knee to the torso and then move it towards the right chest. Use the right hand to help move the left leg. Hold comfortably for 30 seconds. Breathe deeply. Repeat on the right leg. This can be done standing up or lying down. This stretches the piriformis muscle (lower buttock muscle) and external rotators of the hip by internally rotating the hip.

Cat Stretch

Get on your hands and knees on a mat or carpet. Keep your feet together. Press the center of the back upward toward the ceiling. Hold comfortably for 30 seconds. Breathe deeply. Always follow this stretch with a back arch (see next stretch).

Back Arch

Remaining in the hand and knee position from the previous stretch, press the abdomen towards the floor. Do not press the lower abdomen to the floor, otherwise you may place stress on the lower back joints and cause pain or irritation to this region. Hold comfortably for 30 seconds. Breathe deeply. This is an excellent stretch for those who sit all day or have slouching problems.

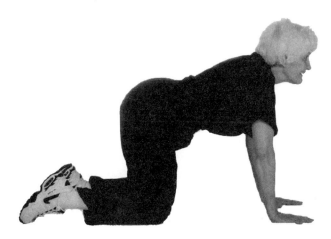

Middle and Low Back Stretches Continued

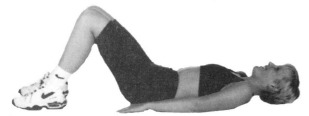

Pelvic Tilt

Lie on your back on the floor with knees bent. Contract the buttocks and press the

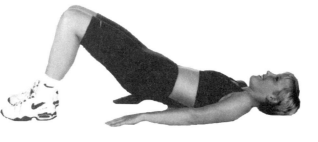

lower back to the floor. This automatically raises the pelvis 1–5 inches off the floor. Do not force this stretch. Let the pelvis rise as naturally as possible. Hold comfortably for 30 seconds. Breathe deeply.

Lying Back Extension

Lie on your stomach. Gently raise the head and upper body off the ground. Support the body with the elbows. Do not arch the back further than it wants to go or you may aggravate any lower back

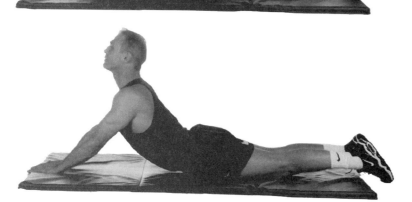

problems that already exist. Hold comfortably for 30 seconds. Breathe deeply. If this causes pain in the low back, buttocks, or legs stop immediately and contact a chiropractor as soon as possible.

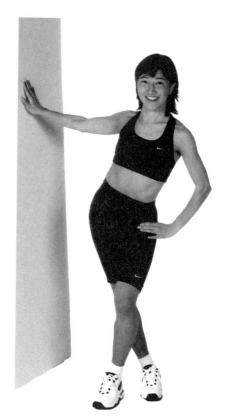

Side of Leg Stretch

Stand approximately 18 inches away from a wall. Use the arm closer to the wall as support against it. Cross the outside leg over the inside leg. Keep the foot of the outside leg flat on the floor. Allow the inside hip to move towards the wall and guide it with a little pressure

Middle and Low Back Stretches Continued

from the outside hand on the outside hip. Keep the spine straight. Hold comfortably for 30 seconds. Breathe deeply. Repeat on the other side. As you become more flexible, you may lean the torso away from the wall, or roll the outside foot so that its bottom faces away from the wall, and hold for 60 seconds to maximize the stretch.

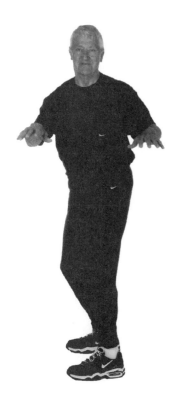

Standing Twist
Keep the feet shoulder-width apart or wider for balance. Slightly bend the knees. Keep

the arms at shoulder level, elbows at 90°, and palms facing the floor. As you twist to the left, turn the neck to the left as well to avoid neck strain. Try to keep the pelvis facing forward and only rotate the spine. Hold comfortably for 30 seconds. Breathe deeply. Twist to the other side.

Sitting Twist (in chair)

Sit with your buttocks against the back of the chair and feet flat on the floor. As you twist the body, grab on to the other side of the chair for stability. Do not force the stretch. Turn the head with the rotation to avoid neck strain. Hold comfortably for 30 seconds. Breathe deeply. You should feel the stretch in the low back and base of the neck. Twist to the other side.

Sitting Twist (on floor)

Sit on the floor with the right leg crossed over the left. Use the right elbow to apply very gentle leverage against the right knee. Rest the left hand on the floor for support. Hold comfortably for 30 seconds. Breathe deeply. Do not use this stretch to crack or adjust the back. This

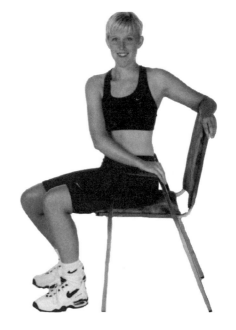

stretch works the buttocks and spinal rotator muscles on the side of the straight leg. Repeat on the other leg.

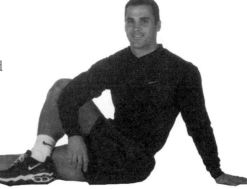

Low Back and Pelvis

Muscles

Piriformis and Tensor fasciae latae (TFL) See page 46.

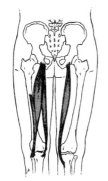

Biceps femoris, Semitendinosus, and Semimembranosus

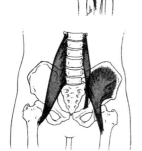

Sartorius and Rectus femoris

Psoas major/minor and Iliacus

Hip muscle problems are associated with 95% of low back syndromes. Any low back or pelvis stretching routine must include stretches that increase flexibility for the hamstring, groin, hip, and inside thigh muscles.

Stretches

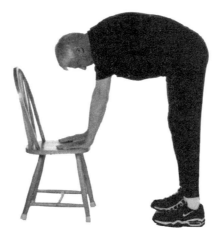

Chair Touch

Stand with the seat of a chair or stool about a foot in front of you. Place the feet shoulder-width apart with knees slightly bent. Bend forward at the waist and use the seat as support. Try to keep the head and neck parallel to the seat. Hold comfortably for 30 seconds. Breathe deeply. If dizziness occurs, consult your chiropractor immediately.

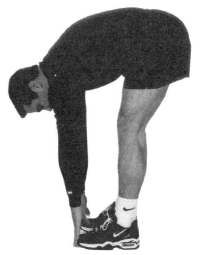

Toe Touch

This stretch is similar to the chair touch stretch. Do this stretch once your flexibility increases to a point where you can comfortably reach the floor. Slightly bend the knees to reduce low back strain. Hold comfortably for 30 seconds. Breathe deeply.

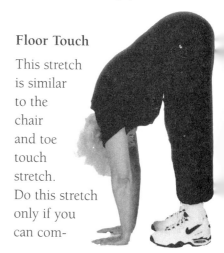

Floor Touch

This stretch is similar to the chair and toe touch stretch. Do this stretch only if you can com-

Low Back and Pelvis Stretches Continued

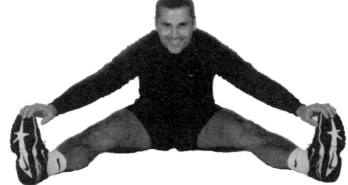

fortably touch the floor with the palm of your hands. Hold comfortably for 30 seconds. Breathe deeply.
(*Note:* Laura, our model, is 70 years old.)

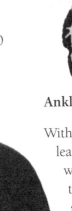

Ankle Reach

With the legs spread apart, lean over the hamstring you wish to stretch. To stretch the inside of the hamstring, lean straight forward. Keep the head up, back straight, and knees slightly bent at all times. Do not round the back. Hold comfortably for 30 seconds. Breathe deeply.

Sitting Toe Touch

Sit on the floor with your feet and legs together and stretched out in front of you. Slowly lean forward until you feel tension in the low back region. Do not lock the knees; keep them slightly bent. Do not force yourself if you cannot touch your toes. Also, do not force your nose to your knees; otherwise, you will strain your neck and upper back. Go as far as you can. Hold comfortably for 30 seconds. Breathe deeply.

One Leg Stretch

Stand close to a chair or wall so that your spine is straight. Hold the foot of the left leg with the left hand and feel the stretch in the front of the thigh. Support yourself with the right hand, if necessary. Hold comfortably for 30 seconds. Breathe deeply. Repeat on the right leg. Avoid using the opposite hand to hold the ankle, because this places a great deal of stress on the knee, shoulder, and neck. Do not lock the knee of the support leg; keep it slightly bent.

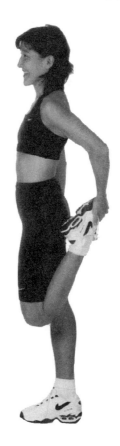

*Low Back and Pelvis Stretches
Continued*

T-Stretch

Hold left ankle with the left hand. Lean body forward so the torso and thigh are approximately parallel to the floor. Keep a slight bend in the support leg, and keep the neck in line with the plane of the body. Hold comfortably for 30 seconds. Breathe deeply. Repeat on the right leg.

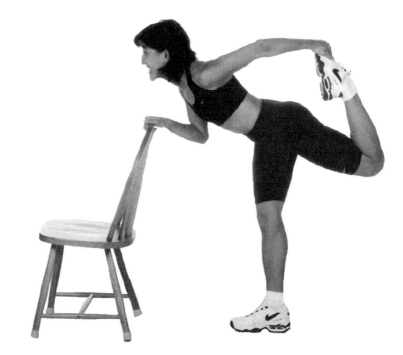

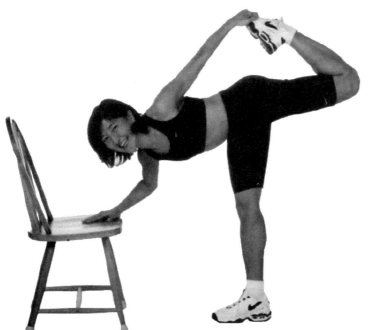

Extreme T-Stretch
This is the same as the T-stretch, except as the hip becomes more flexible, you may be able to raise the leg higher. Do not arch the back during this stretch. Hold comfortably for 30 seconds. Breathe deeply. Repeat on the other side.

Low Back and Pelvis Stretches Continued

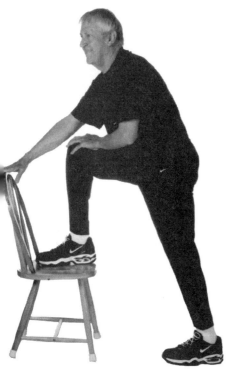

Standing Hip Stretch

Keep the spine straight with a slight lean forward. Keep the top of the left foot on a chair seat, bench, or box. Support yourself with your right hand (or both hands) on the back of another chair or against a wall. Lean slightly forward. Feel the stretch in the front of the hip on the back leg. Hold for 30 seconds. Breathe deeply. Repeat on the other side.

Chair Lunge

Using a chair or a box, place one foot flat on the chair seat or box. Keep the spine straight. Gently push the pelvis forward and feel the stretch in the front of the hip region on the back leg. Hold comfortably for 30 seconds. Breathe deeply. This is an excellent and safe stretch for seniors or pregnant women. Repeat on the other side.

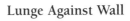

Lunge Against Wall

Keep the spine straight, head raised, and palms against a wall for support. Bend the front knee 90° and keep the foot flat on the ground. If possible, rest the rear knee gently on the floor to prevent bouncing during the stretch. Keep the rear ankle bent to help support you. Press the pelvis toward the wall. Feel the stretch at the front hip of the back leg. Hold comfortably for 30 seconds. Breathe deeply. Repeat on the other side.

Low Back and Pelvis Stretches Continued

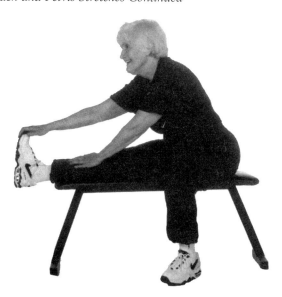

Seated Hamstring Stretch

Place one leg on a bench in front of you. The opposite foot should rest flat on the floor with the knee bent for optimum control of the stretch. Bend at the waist while keeping the neck and back straight. Slowly lean the upper torso forward. Never touch the nose to the knee (rounded back); otherwise, it puts too much stresses on the upper back and neck. Hold comfortably for 30 seconds. Breathe deeply. Repeat on the other leg.

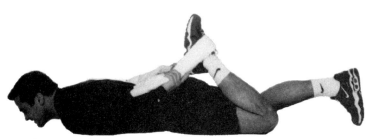

Towel-Assisted Thigh Stretch

If you are unable to reach the ankle (as in the one leg stretch, see p. 51), use a towel to help you. You can hold it with one hand and support yourself on the floor with the other. Or you can hold the towel with both hands and rest your forehead on a pillow. Hold comfortably for 30 seconds. Repeat on the other side.

The Abdominal Region

Front Abdomen

Muscles

Psoas major/minor and Iliacus See page 50.

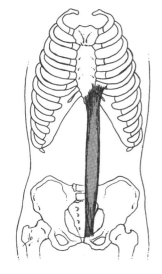

Rectus abdominis

Stretches

Back Arch
See page 47.

Lying Back Extension
See page 48.

T-Stretch
See page 52.

Extreme T-Stretch
See page 52.

Chair Lunge
See page 53.

Standing Hip Stretch
See page 53.

Lunge Against Wall
See page 53.

Tall Stretch
See page 37.

Side of Abdomen

Muscles

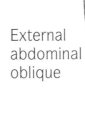

External abdominal oblique

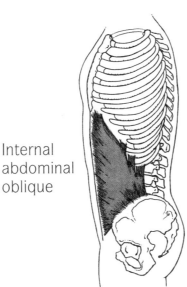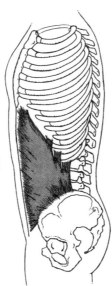

Internal abdominal oblique

Stretches

Standing Twist
See page 49.

Sitting Twist (in chair)
See page 49.

Sitting Twist (on floor)
See page 49.

Standing Lateral Bend
See page 37.

Sitting Lateral Bend
See page 38.

Case Study #6: Acute Abdominal Pain

History: L.N., a 29-year-old bartender, had acute right-side stomach pain for 3 weeks. The pain caused by her to limp. She also had low back pain for 2 years.

Diagnosis: Right stomach pain and limp were caused by nerve irritation from the vertebra and pelvis.

Treatment: Spinal adjustment, massage, and stretching.

Result: Immediate reduction of stomach pain.

Note: *No recurrence of stomach pain in the last 6 months.*

The Thigh

Front of Thigh Muscles

Psoas and Iliacus
See page 50.

Sartorius and Rectus femoris
See page 50.

Stretches

One Leg Stretch
See page 51.

T-Stretch
See page 52.

Extreme T-Stretch
See page 52.

Chair Lunge
See page 53.

Standing Thigh (Hip) Stretch
See page 53.

Lunge Against Wall
See page 53.

Inner Thigh Muscles

Psoas and Iliacus
See page 50.

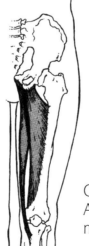

Gracilis and Adductor magnus

Stretches

Side Lunge

Stand with feet wider than shoulder-width apart. Point toes slightly outward. Keep the feet flat on the floor and balance yourself by placing your hands on your thighs. Bend one knee and slowly move the body to that side. Do not lean forward. Hold comfortably for 30 seconds. Breathe deeply. This will stretch the opposite groin. Lean to the other side.

Inner Thigh Stretches Continued

Supine Groin Stretch

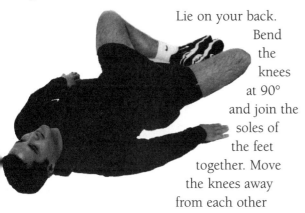

Lie on your back. Bend the knees at 90° and join the soles of the feet together. Move the knees away from each other towards the floor. Hold comfortably for 30 seconds. Breathe deeply. If you feel undue stress in the groin or hip area, place a pillow under each knee to minimize the stress.

Wall Groin Stretch

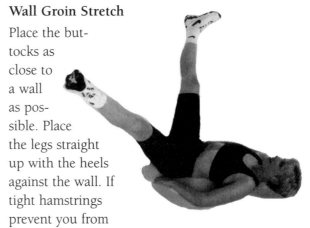

Place the buttocks as close to a wall as possible. Place the legs straight up with the heels against the wall. If tight hamstrings prevent you from touching the wall, move in as close as possible. Keep both arms out on the floor for support. Slowly separate the legs until you feel a slight pain in the groin. Then bring the legs back up about ¼ inch. Hold comfortably for 30 seconds. Breathe deeply. Avoid this stretch if you have had a previous hip injury.

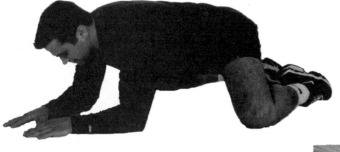

Prone Groin Stretch
Separate the knees and drop to your elbows. The spine will slope downwards to the floor. Try to keep the head and neck straight so that the forehead rests gently on the floor or on a pillow. Do not arch the back. Feel the stretch inside the thigh. Hold comfortably for 30 seconds. Breathe deeply. This stretch is also called the "hockey stretch."

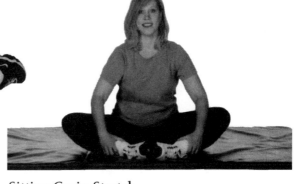

Sitting Groin Stretch
Sit on the floor with the back straight, soles of the feet together, and knees apart. Separate the knees towards the floor. Do not force the knees to touch the floor. Use the hands and arms to hold the legs in one position during the stretch. If needed, you can lean forward slightly with elbows on knees to further your stretch. Do not bounce. Hold for 30–60 seconds for optimal stretch. Breathe deeply.

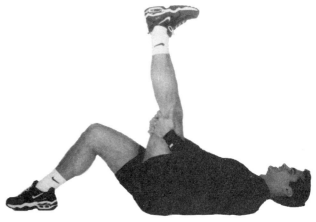

Outer Thigh
Muscles

Piriformis and Tensor Fasciae Latae (TFL)
See page 46.

Stretch

Side of Leg Stretch
See page 48.

Back of Thigh
Muscles

Hamstring Group: Biceps femoris, Semitendinosus, and Semimembranosus
See page 50.

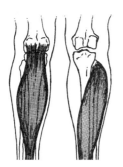

Calf Group: Gastrocnemius and Soleus

Stretches

Chair Touch
See page 50.

Toe Touch
See page 50.

Floor Touch
See page 50.

Sitting Toe Touch
See page 51.

Ankle Reach
See page 51.

Seated Hamstring Stretch
See page 54.

Lying Hamstring Stretch

Try this stretch only if you have easily progressed through the previous hamstring stretches, or if you can raise your legs straight up at 90°. Lie on the floor and raise one leg up 90°. Bend the opposite knee at 90° to reduce stress on the low back. Clasp both hands either: 1) above the knee to stretch the entire hamstring; 2) below the knee to stretch upper hamstring at pelvis.

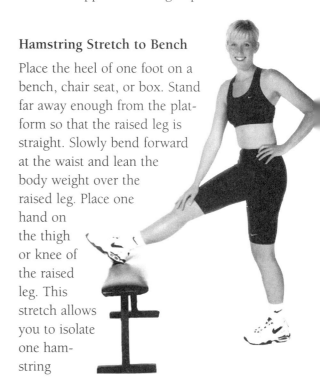

Hamstring Stretch to Bench

Place the heel of one foot on a bench, chair seat, or box. Stand far away enough from the platform so that the raised leg is straight. Slowly bend forward at the waist and lean the body weight over the raised leg. Place one hand on the thigh or knee of the raised leg. This stretch allows you to isolate one hamstring

Back of Thigh Stretches Continued

at a time. Never round the back as you lean forward. Hold comfortably for 30 seconds. Breathe deeply. Repeat with the other leg.

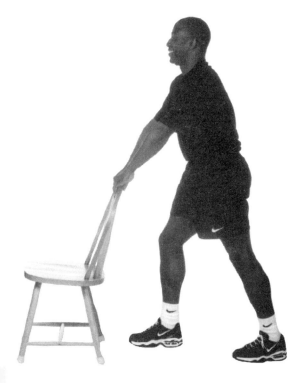

Straight Leg Stretch

Place hands on the back of a chair or against a wall for support. Keep the front knee bent with the shin straight. Keep both feet flat on the floor and the spine straight. Keeping the back leg straight, slide it back until you feel the stretch in the back of the lower leg behind the knee. Hold comfortably for 30–60 seconds. Breathe deeply. Repeat with the other leg. This stretches the muscle that runs down the back of the leg to form the Achilles' tendon at the heel.

Note: Muscles that are more fibrous, such as tendons, require more time (30–60 seconds) to effectively stretch.

Front of the Lower Leg/Calf Region

Muscles

Extensor digitorum,
Tibialis anterior,
Extensor hallucis

Stretches

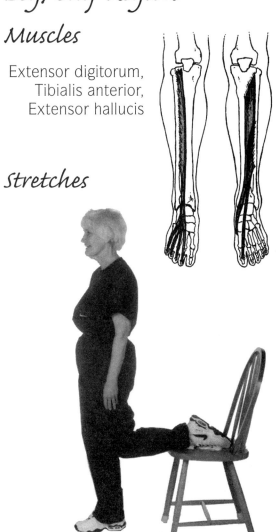

Standing Shin Stretch

Rest the top of one foot on the seat of a chair or on a box so that the knee is bent at 90°. For a deeper stretch, press down on the heel of the back leg with the hand of the same side. Hold for 30 seconds. Breathe deeply. Repeat with the other leg.

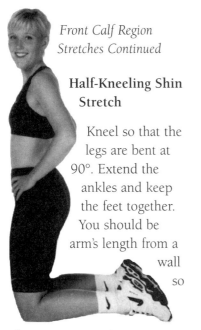

Front Calf Region Stretches Continued

Half-Kneeling Shin Stretch

Kneel so that the legs are bent at 90°. Extend the ankles and keep the feet together. You should be arm's length from a wall so that you can use it as support, if needed. Do not sit back; otherwise, it will strain your knees. Hold for 30 seconds. Breathe deeply.

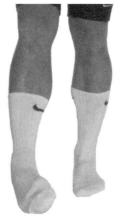

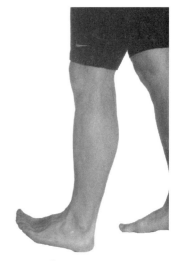

Outer Ankle Stretch

While standing or sitting, point the toes of one foot, straighten the ankle, and then point inward to stretch the outer ankle. Hold for 30–40 seconds. Breathe deeply. Repeat with the other ankle.

Toe Extending

Sit comfortably on a chair and place the heel of one foot on the floor. Point the toes upward to stretch the arch muscles of the foot. Hold for 30 seconds. Breathe deeply. Repeat with the other foot.

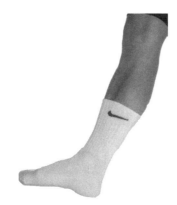

Inner Ankle Stretch

While standing or sitting, point the toes of one foot, straighten the ankle, and then point outward to stretch the inner ankle. Hold for 30–40 seconds. Breathe deeply. Repeat with the other ankle.

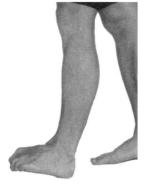

Toe Flexing

Sit comfortably on a chair and place the heel of one foot on the floor. Point the toes downward to contract the arch muscles and stretch the top of the foot and toes. Hold for 30 seconds. Breathe deeply. Repeat with the other foot.

Back of Lower Leg/Calf Region

Muscles

Calf Group:
Gastrocnemius and
Soleus See page 58.

Stretches

Straight Leg Stretch
See page 59.

Toe Extending
See page 60.

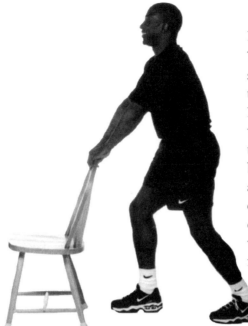

Bent-Knee Calf Stretch

This stretch is similar to the straight leg stretch except that the back leg is slightly bent. Perform the straight leg stretch until you feel a mild stretch in the calf of the back leg. Then bend the knee of the back leg about 5° to stretch the deeper calf muscles. Hold for 30 seconds. Breathe deeply. Repeat with the other leg. This stretch is also called a "soleus stretch."

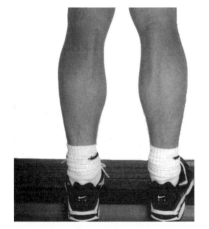

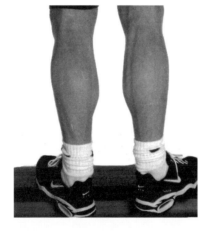

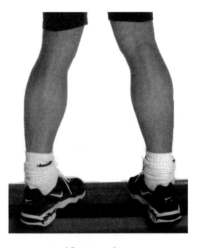

Calf Stretch on a Step

Use the railing and wall for support as you place the front half of the feet on a step. Prop the heels below the step. Keep the knees slightly bent for a deep calf muscle stretch or straight for an outer calf muscle stretch. Hold comfortably for 30 seconds. Breathe deeply.

Inner Calf Stretch

This stretch is similar to the calf stretch on a step, except, with the toes out, you stretch the inner calf muscles. Hold comfortably for 30 seconds. Breathe deeply.

Outer Calf Stretch

This stretch is similar to the calf stretch on a step, except, with the toes in, you stretch the outer calf muscles. Hold comfortably for 30 seconds. Breathe deeply.

Outside of Lower Leg/Calf Region

Muscles

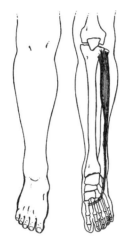

Peroneus longus

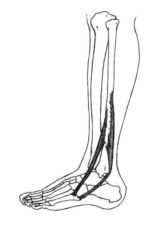

Peroneus brevis/
tertius

Stretch

Outer Ankle Stretch
See page 60.

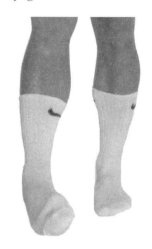

The Daily Shower Stretch Routine

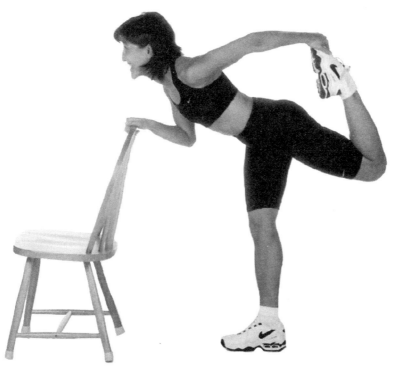

A daily 10–15 minute stretch routine can get your body ready to attack each day and put forth 110% in all you do. The deep breathing involved also gives you the opportunity to meditate and mentally prepare yourself for your daily events. The shower is the perfect place to perform your routine. In addition to gaining flexibility, the warm water helps the muscles relax and lengthen because it increases circulation.

The massaging effect of the water also helps override the muscles' protective stretch reflex so that you can get into the strengthening or relaxing part of the stretch faster.

The bending and turning movements that we all perform in the shower will prepare your muscles for stretching, just like walking in place before stretching helps improves circulation. The shower stretch routine allows you to warm up by washing your body first. It is also an effective routine because it is easy and becomes a habit. Showering every day will remind you to stretch every day. Chapter 2 describes other possible times and places to stretch if, for instance, you take baths instead, or if your shower can become slippery and you prefer to stretch somewhere more stable. You can do all of these stretches anywhere you wish. The point is to do it regularly, every day.

SHOWER STRETCH ROUTINE

Remember the Six Rules to Stretching
(see Chapter 6) when doing this routine.

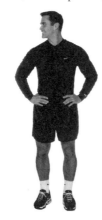
See page 32.

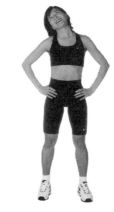
See page 31.

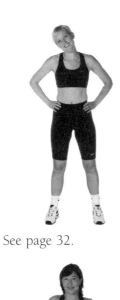
See page 33.

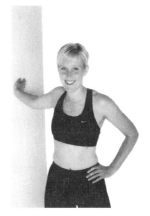
See page 38.

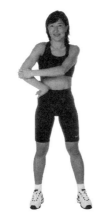
See page 36.

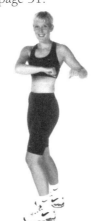
See page 49.

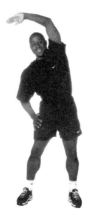
See page 37.

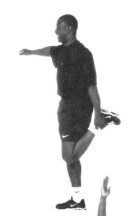
See page 51.

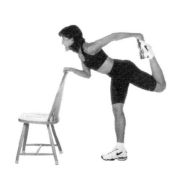
See page 52.

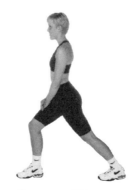
See page 59.

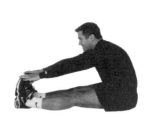
See page 51.

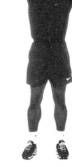
See page 37.

SENIOR'S DAILY STRETCH ROUTINE

This series of stretches is particularly gentle and effective for seniors. It too can be done in the shower, or anywhere. Remember to follow the Six Rules to Stretching (see Chapter 6).

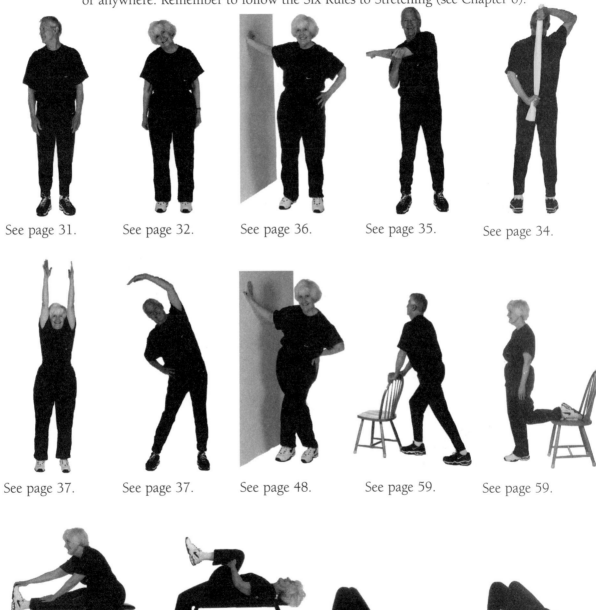

See page 31.   See page 32.   See page 36.   See page 35.   See page 34.

See page 37.   See page 37.   See page 48.   See page 59.   See page 59.

See page 54.   See page 46.   See page 48.   See page 48.

STRETCHES FOR TRAVELING

Vacation time affects our daily routines, including stretching. But there are many reasons why you shouldn't forget to stretch while traveling. First, sitting for long periods of time significantly tightens the front hip flexors, low back muscles, hamstrings, calves, front neck muscles, and shoulders. This is because most travel seats are L-shaped and have no spinal curved support, which can cause muscles to stiffen up quickly. A good way to correct the seating is to place one regular pillow or two small ones behind the back, about 4 inches above the waist. This will maintain the normal curves of the spine as well as reduce back, shoulder, and neck tension. Second, sleeping on different beds with various pillows can cause strain to the muscular system. For these reasons, stretching will keep you limber and prepared for all the activities ahead so that you can enjoy your vacation to the fullest.

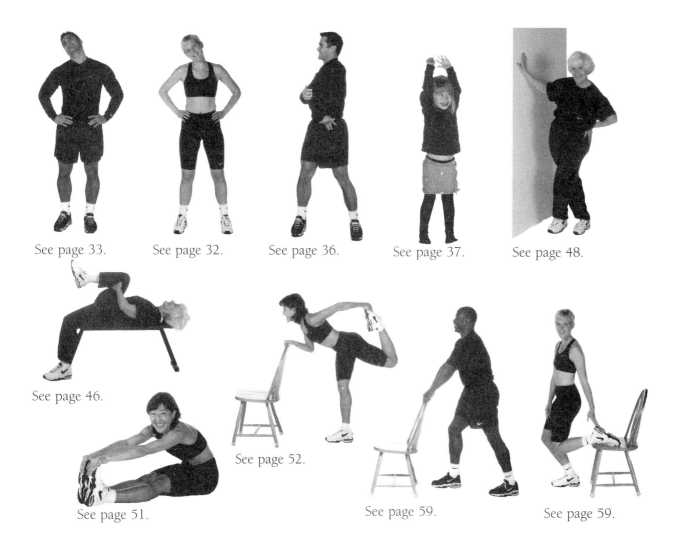

See page 33.   See page 32.   See page 36.   See page 37.   See page 48.

See page 46.

See page 51.

See page 52.

See page 59.

See page 59.

Dangerous & Harmful Movements

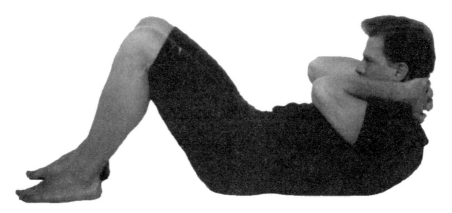

*R*esearch done today has shown that the majority of popular stretch/exercise manuals and videos contain many movements that can actually injure you. They can strain underlying joints, nerves, ligaments, and muscle tissues. Much time and effort was put into this book to ensure that you are provided with a safe and useful guide of proper methods for increasing flexibility. At this time, we want to show you what *not* to do when beginning a stretch, exercise, or flexibility program.

While creating this chapter, we reviewed many popular stretch/yoga/exercise videos and books currently on the market. Some moves in these instructional aids are not only inappropriate but they also neglect to follow the Six Rules to Stretching in Chapter 6. You should avoid the moves in this chapter, even if they are in your favorite video or class (i.e., yoga or aerobics). If you have been doing some of them for years, we suggest that you not do them anymore. They can actually limit your ability to stretch/exercise as well as damage important joints and ligaments. On the other hand, if your video or class does contain safe stretches (as discussed in Chapter 7), but does not follow the Six Rules to Stretching (i.e., holding the stretch for 30 seconds, being gentle, breathing, etc.), simply incorporate them into your stretching.

Every position deemed harmful (thirty-four in total) is shown in this chapter with a brief explanation of which parts of the body can be strained by doing it. You can then understand why certain regions of the body become injured or reinjured by doing these inappropriate moves. It would also be a good idea to refer to Chapter 7 to see the anatomy behind each movement and see for yourself why they are not designed for any specific muscle or specific direction of any muscle fibers.

Remember, the goal of any fitness routine is to maximize the benefits to the body without causing any harm. Through our years of biomechanical expertise and experience, we hope that pointing out these harmful movements to you will help steer you to a better path. Some of these are sure to surprise you.

Extreme Neck Extension

This stretch strains the joints of the neck, which can lead to compression of the nerves and arteries along the neck. The result can be pain and even dizziness. There have been reported cases of stroke after prolonged extension of the neck. People mostly assume this position at the hairdresser's. Try to avoid it.

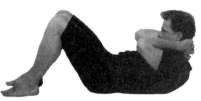

Crunches

The back of the neck, shoulders, and upper back muscles are strained, which can cause dizziness, headaches, and numbness in the arms and hands. If you have neck or shoulder tension, avoid this move. It is our view that the risk of a strained neck outweighs the reward of a toned stomach.

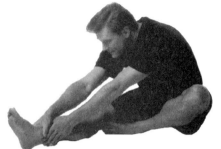

Foot into Groin Hamstring Stretch

This commonly causes a great deal of strain to the low back and pelvic joint of the side of the bent knee. Additionally, bending forward will significantly stress the neck and upper back muscles.

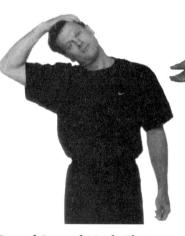

Forced Lateral Neck Flexion

This strains or can even tear the neck muscles by overstretching the ligaments opposite to where the head is tilting. The muscle contracts, as opposed to stretches, to protect itself.

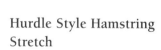

Crunches with Twist

This exercise can cause the same type of strain as does regular crunches. Here the twisting motion adds stress to the spine. Avoid this stretch if you suffer from frequent headaches. It will aggravate the condition.

Hurdle Style Hamstring Stretch

This hurdle style stretch aggravates the knees and hip joints.

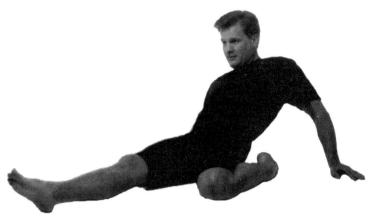

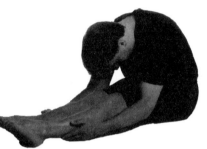

Leaning Back Hurdle Position

This position places the same kind of strain as the hurdle style stretch. In addition, it strains the lower back and neck.

Nose to Knee Stretch

This position places a great deal of strain on the neck and shoulders.

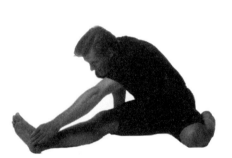

Leaning Forward Hurdle Position

This causes strain to the same areas as the leaning back hurdle position.

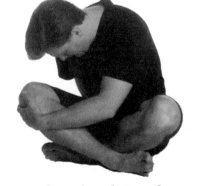

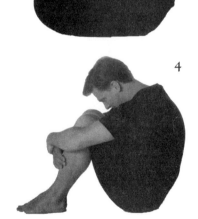

Cross-legged Back Stretch

This strains the hip joint on the side opposite of the head tilt. This also stresses the neck, shoulder, and upper back.

Back Roll

Many people do this to stretch the spine, but it strains the neck and shoulder area.

Lying Forced Spinal Hyperextension

This stretch jams the spinal joints, from the top to the bottom.

Inverted and Modified Inverted Pike

This causes the same strains as the shoulder stand. But, because of the forward position of the legs, there is more strain on the neck and shoulders.

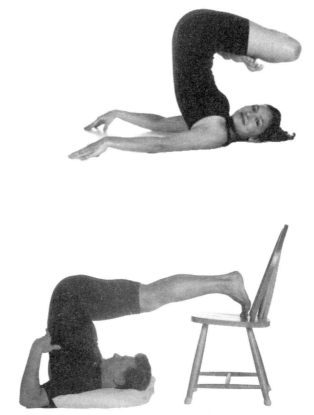

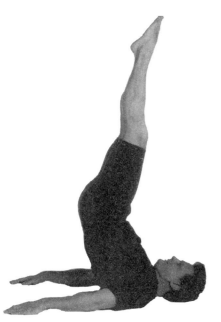

Shoulder Stand
This stretch is done in yoga, but it puts excessive strain on the neck and upper back joints and ligaments.

Legs over Head

This stretch causes an even greater strain on the neck than the inverted pike stretch. It is one of the most dangerous postures that we have come across.

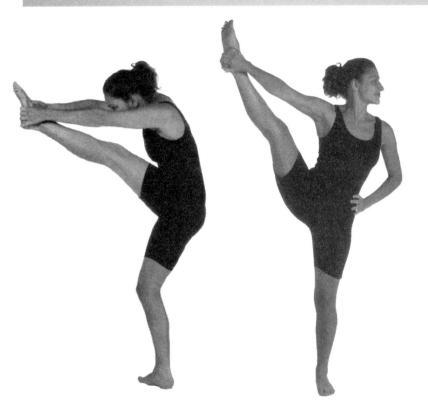

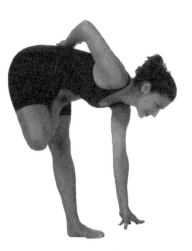

Bent Over Figure 4
This stretch causes hip, knees, and lower back strain.

Standing and Modified Standing Bound Half Lotus Position
The hamstring of the raised leg is strained as well as the neck.

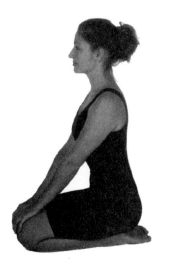

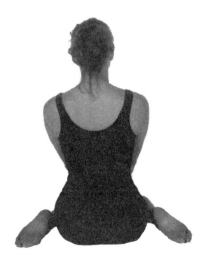

**Double-knee Crush
(Side and Back View)**

Small children are often seen sitting this way. It should be avoided by everyone because it causes strain to the knee ligament and tendon. It also causes compression on the blood vessels in the back of the legs, particularly the knee joints.

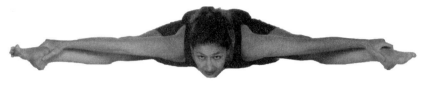

Seated Angled Posture

Doing this stretch puts strain on the groin, leg muscles, and neck.

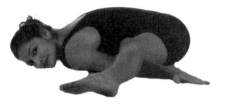

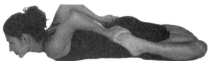

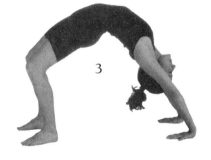

Frog Position

This stretch strains the knee joints and muscles as well as the neck.

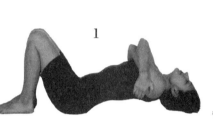

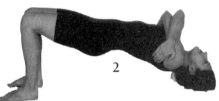

Bridge and Modified Bridge Posture

The three steps to this stretch cause strain on the shoulder and neck joints. The final stance compresses the mid and lower back joints. Children under the age of 16 should not do this stretch in gymnastics class because their bones are not fully formed yet and, thus, they are prone to injury.

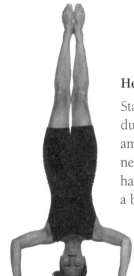

Head Stand

Standing on your head produces a tremendous amount of pressure on the neck joints and discs. A handstand against a wall is a better position to assume.

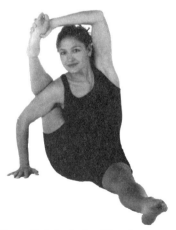

Foot Behind the Head Posture

This stretch strains the hip joint and neck.

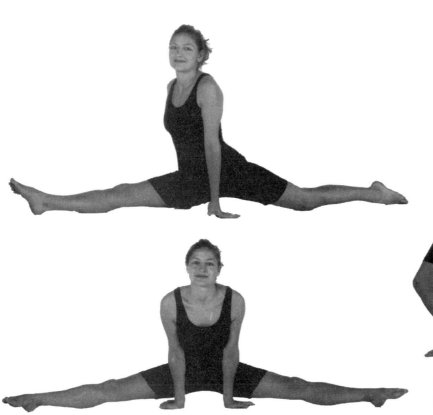

Warrior Position of the Sun Salutation Series

This stretch strains the lower back and compresses the joints of the lower neck if done incorrectly. However, if you press your head and lower back gently upward and backward, it is safe.

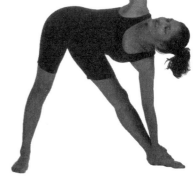

Side and Forward Split

Through supervision, time, and practice, you can train yourself to do these moves without harm. However, a beginner should not immediately try to force these positions. Whichever direction the torso faces, this stretch strains the groin, pelvis, hips, and the ligaments in the knees.

Revolved Triangle Posture

This is very dangerous to the joints, ligaments, and spinal discs of the lower back. The lower back is not meant to bend and twist like this. Many people trying this stretch have hurt themselves.

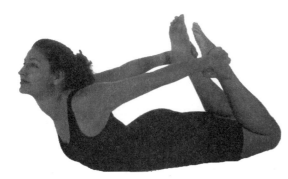

Bow Posture

Curling the body backward strains the neck, lower back, front shoulders, knees, and ankles.

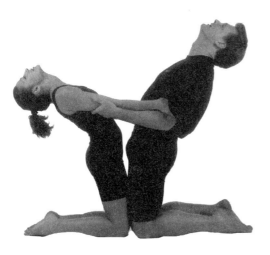

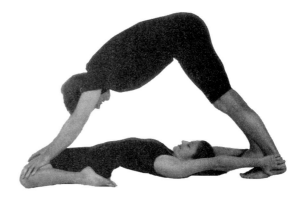

Dynamic Body Extension

This stretch can strain the lower back and jam the neck joints unless you press your head and lower back gently up and back as in the Warrior Position of the Sun Salutation Series.

Partner Assisted Double Knee Crush

The person on the bottom risks serious knee joint and ligament damage.

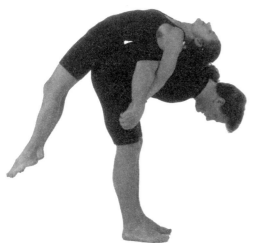

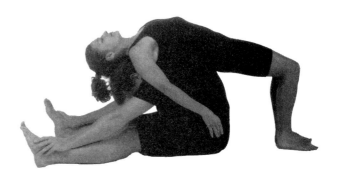

Partner Assisted Spinal Flexion and Hamstring Stretch

The person on the bottom risks straining the lower back, neck, shoulders, and hamstring.

Spinal Extension Using Gravity and a Partner

The person underneath risks straining the discs of the lower back as well as the blood vessels of the neck and head. The person on top risks jamming the spinal joints and thus compressing the nerves. Some people use this technique to try to manipulate their own spinal joints. It is very *non*-specific and could easily hurt rather than help the spine.

Stretches for Specific Sports

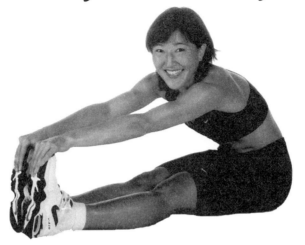

*I*n this chapter, individual stretches have been selected to give practical and safe stretch routines for specific sports. They will help improve your performance and decrease the risk of injury.

The stress of exercise or competition can be a positive one. In fact, stress is defined as any stimulus that causes the body to change in order to adapt to that particular stress. A positive stress, or eustress, stimulates the body to make changes that improve health and well-being, such as decreased heart rate, lowered cholesterol, and improved lung capacity. In order for the body to maintain or improve its function, it must receive eustress regularly. By properly preparing for stress by stretching, we can maximize its positive effects and minimize its negative effects.

However, too much of a good thing is not so good. For example, if you exercise too much, or overtrain, the body cannot adapt if it is too great. This can lead to breakdowns, such as injury, tiredness, weight loss, decreased enthusiasm, and so on. Overtraining can be in the form of one large insult or many small traumas called "microtraumas." The body is unable to detect or deal

with many of the microtraumas that happen if work intensity and frequency are too high. In order for the athlete to keep pushing the body to new limits, certain aspects of his or her lifestyle must be addressed, such as proper diet, rest, and being physically and psychologically prepared. The quintessential element of preparation is stretching.

Being fit does not necessarily mean being healthy. Working the body to a higher level, especially when the training is geared towards one repetitive movement, requires that you take even greater care of your body. Increasing the range of motion is the goal when designing a sports-specific stretch routine to maximize performance. Range of motion is divided into two main types:

1. Intrinsic: These include the joints and ligaments. Chiropractic adjustments can alter these in a positive way, while injury can alter them in a negative way.

2. Extrinsic: These are the *voluntary* movements around a joint actively governed by muscles and tendons. Although you can mostly control your muscles, they frequently shorten on their own either through some form of injury, poor posture, lack of use, or as part of a protective reflex (such as a spasm). Stretching and strength-training exercises are for altering this area.

It is only when both the intrinsic and extrinsic ranges of motion are working that you can begin to maximize your flexibility. This chapter concentrates on improving extrinsic motion in relation to the activity. The stretches are based on the understanding of the key movements of each sport.

Scientific literature reviewed emphasizes that the length of the stretch routine, including the warm-up, should be 15–20% of the total exercise time (see p. 9). For example, a 60-minute workout should start with 12 minutes of stretching after the warm-up. This decreases the chance of injury as well as increases strength and effectiveness of the training.

Equally important as the warm-up is the cool-down. For an hour of exercise, you should spend 3–6 minutes relaxing and stretching the muscles that specifically relate to the activity. This will substantially reduce the pain, stiffness, and buildup of waste (see pages 9–10).

Note: Remember always to follow the Six Rules to Stretching (see Chapter 6). As you perform each stretch, emphasize the muscles you will use in the sport or activity.

Facts

1. Athletes must be flexible, pliable, malleable, and adaptable. If they are too rigid or tight, they are much more likely to become injured.
2. Most sports injuries are caused by structural and muscular imbalances.
3. Injuries, although uncomfortable, are the most efficient way your body gets your attention.

THE STRETCHES FOR EACH SPORT

The four general stretches below should be a mandatory part of every stretch routine you do. Ideally, all the stretches listed for each specific sport in this chapter should be done *in the order shown* before and after the activity. However, if you are in a rush, you should do at least these four before the sport and the ones asterisked (*) afterwards.

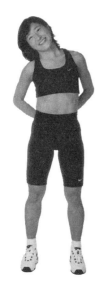

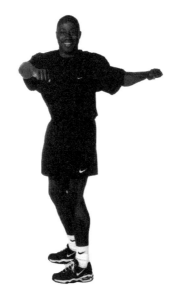

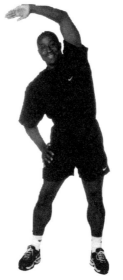

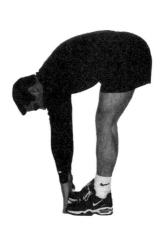

See page 32.   See page 49.   See page 37.   See page 50.

Alpine (Downhill) Skiing

Skiers are prone to equipment-related injuries. Wearing boots that are too consistently tight may create enough pressure to damage the nerve running from the knee to the foot. The same nerve may be damaged at the knee by the persistent stress of sharp turns.

Most Common Injuries: Knee sprain and strain; ligament tear; neck hyperextension; wrist sprain; finger sprain and fracture.

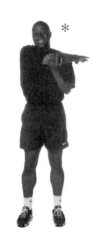

See page 35.

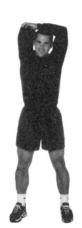

See page 36.

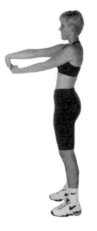

See page 44.

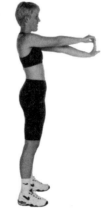

See page 44.

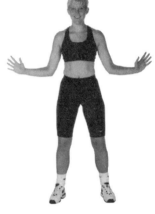

See page 43.

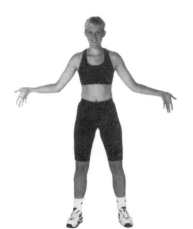

See page 43.

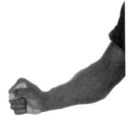

See page 44.

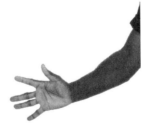

See page 44.

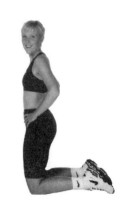

See page 60.

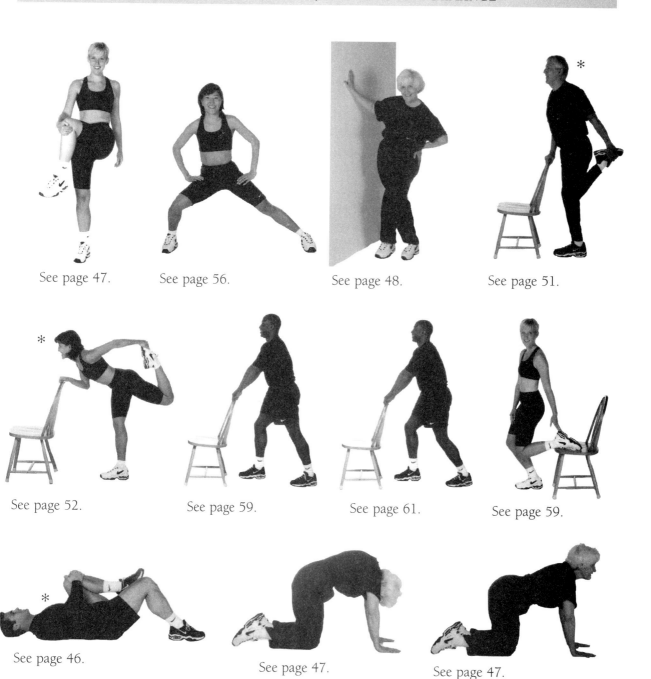

See page 47.   See page 56.   See page 48.   See page 51.

See page 52.   See page 59.   See page 61.   See page 59.

See page 46.   See page 47.   See page 47.

Badminton

Most Common Injuries: Ankle sprain; hamstring strain; wrist/elbow strain; low back strain.

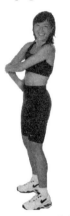

See page 31.

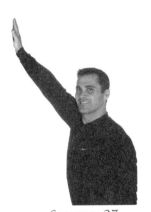

See page 33.

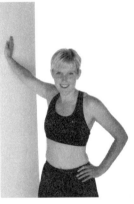

See page 35.

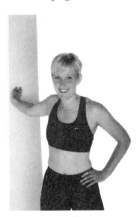

See page 36.

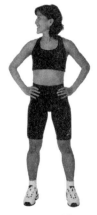

See page 36.

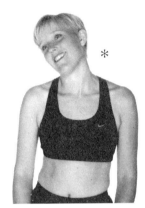

See page 37.

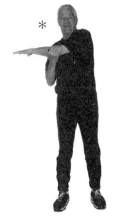

See page 36.

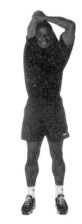

See page 38.

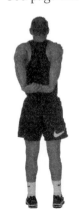

See page 40.

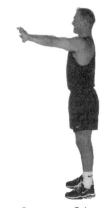

See page 34.

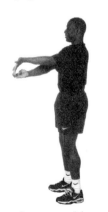

See page 44.

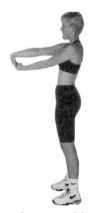

See page 44.

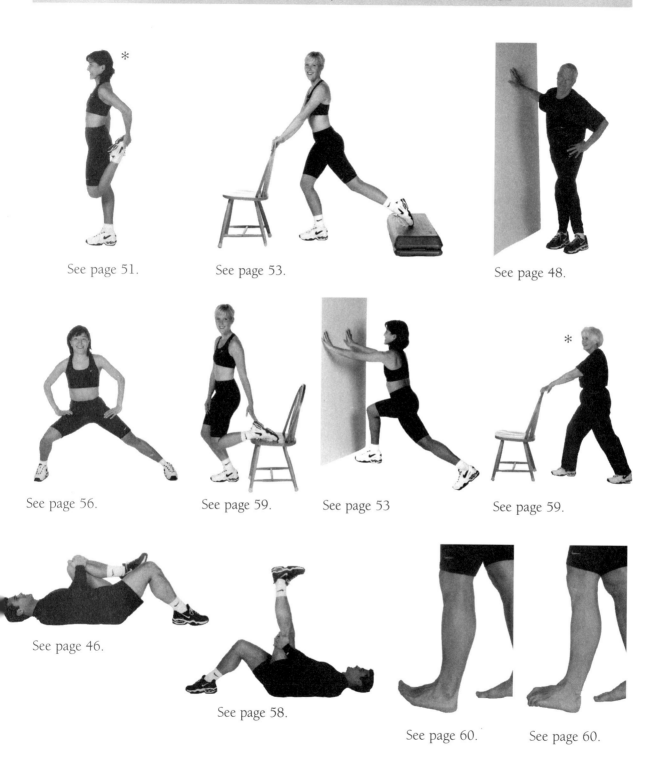

See page 51.

See page 53.

See page 48.

See page 56.

See page 59.

See page 53

See page 59.

See page 46.

See page 58.

See page 60.

See page 60.

Baseball/Cricket

Baseball requires an overhead throwing motion that tends to pull and damage the main nerves from the neck through the shoulder to cause muscle weakness. Pitchers can suffer damage to the elbow region, or funny bone, which results in pain, tingling, and weakness in the forearm and hand. A Japanese study revealed that nerve injuries happen most often to mountain climbers, gymnasts, and baseball players.

Most Common Injuries: Rotator cuff (shoulder) strain; low back strain or sprain; hamstring, calf, neck, elbow, and wrist strain.

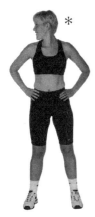

See page 31.

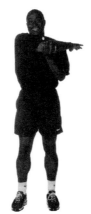

See page 35.

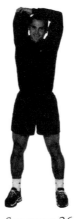

See page 36.

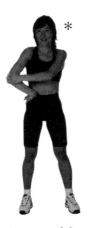

See page 36.

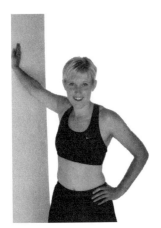

See page 36.

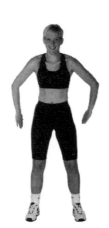

See page 35.

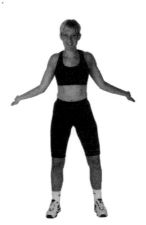

See page 39.

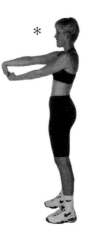

See page 44.

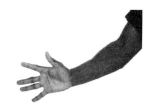

See page 44.

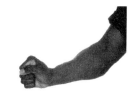

See page 44.

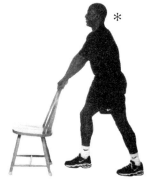
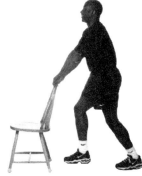

See page 59.

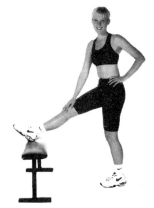

See page 61.

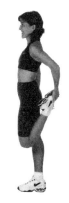

See page 51.

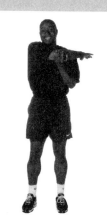

See page 58.

Basketball/Volleyball

Most Common Injuries: Finger strain/sprain/fracture; wrist sprain; hamstring and calf strain; ankle and knee ligament sprain; shoulder strain; neck strain/sprain.

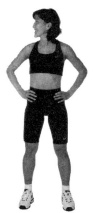

See page 31.

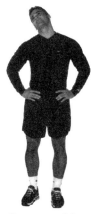

See page 33.

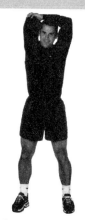

See page 35.

See page 36.

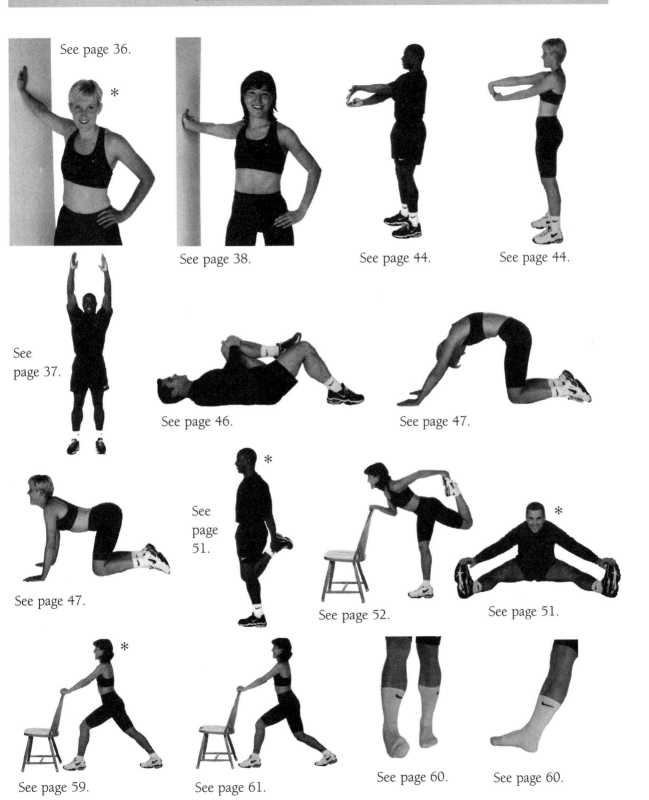

See page 36.

See page 38.

See page 44.

See page 44.

See page 37.

See page 46.

See page 47.

See page 47.

See page 51.

See page 52.

See page 51.

See page 59.

See page 61.

See page 60.

See page 60.

83

Boxing/Cardio Kick-Boxing

Most Common Injuries: Concussion; knee strain/sprain; shoulder strain; bicep spasm; finger sprain/dislocation; wrist sprain; rib strain/sprain/fracture.

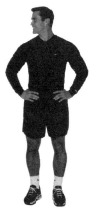

See page 31.

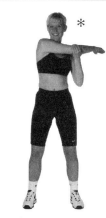

*

See page 33.

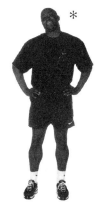

*

See page 35.

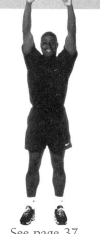

See page 37.

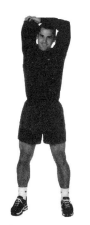

See page 36.

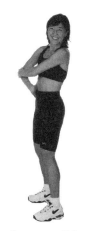

See page 36.

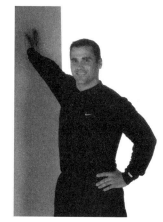

See page 36.

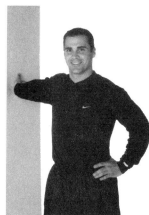

See page 38.

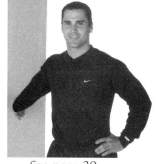

See page 39.

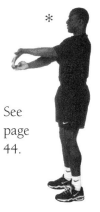

*

See page 44.

See page 44.

See page 51.

84

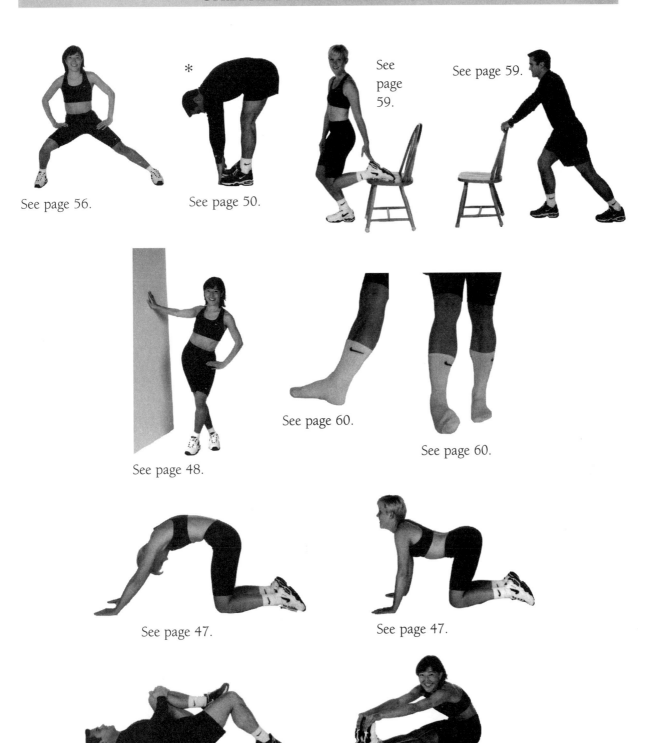

See page 56.

*

See page 50.

See page 59.

See page 59.

See page 48.

See page 60.

See page 60.

See page 47.

See page 47.

See page 46.

See page 51.

Canoeing/Kayaking

Most Common Injuries: Shoulder (rotator cuff), neck, and spinal strain.

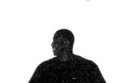
See page 31.

*
See page 33.

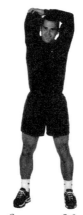
See page 36.

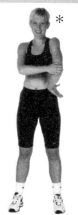
*
See page 36.

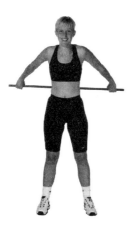
See page 40.

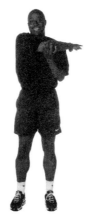
See page 35.

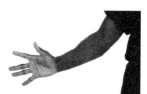
See page 44.

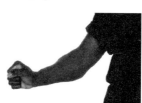
See page 44.

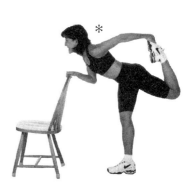
*
See page 52.

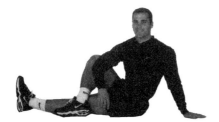
See page 49.

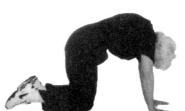
See page 47.

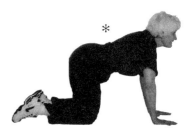
*
See page 47.

Climbing

It is often the equipment rather than the climb that causes problems. Heavy backpacks can put damaging pressure on the neck and shoulder nerves, leading to numbness and weakness in the arms.

Most Common Injuries: Finger and wrist strain; calf spasm; mid and low back strain; shoulder dislocation; general fractures.

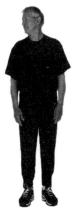
See page 31.

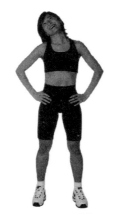
See page 33.

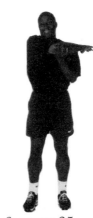
See page 35.

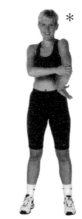
See page 36.

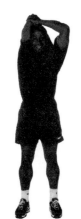
See page 36.

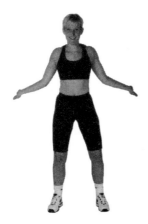
See page 39.

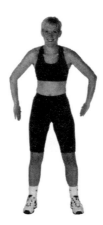
See page 35.

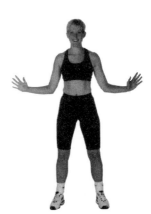
See page 43.

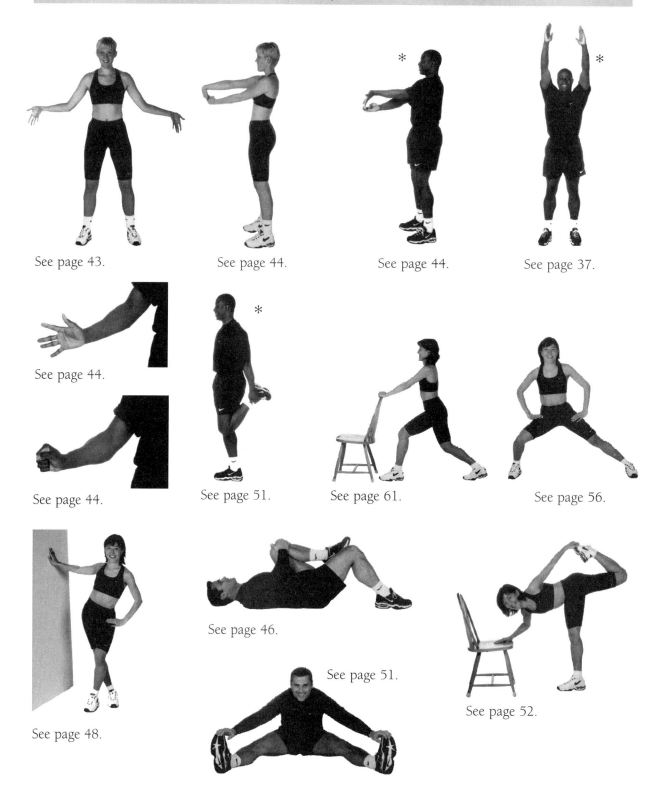

See page 43.

See page 44.

*

See page 44.

*

See page 37.

See page 44.

See page 44.

*

See page 51.

See page 61.

See page 56.

See page 48.

See page 46.

See page 51.

See page 52.

See page 47.

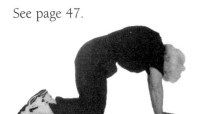

See page 47.

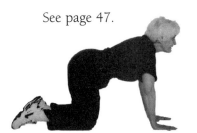

See page 60.

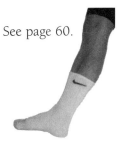

Curling

Most Common Injuries: Hip and shoulder strain; pelvic joint blockage.

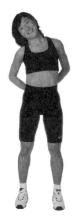

See page 32.

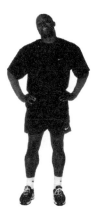

See page 33.

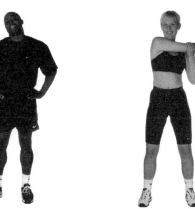

See page 35.

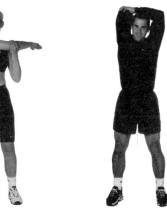

See page 36.

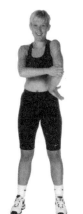

See page 36.

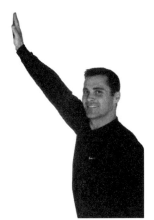

See page 37.

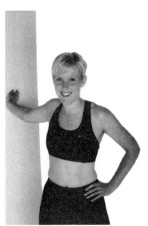

See page 38.

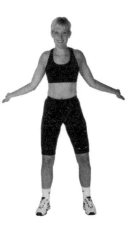

See page 39.

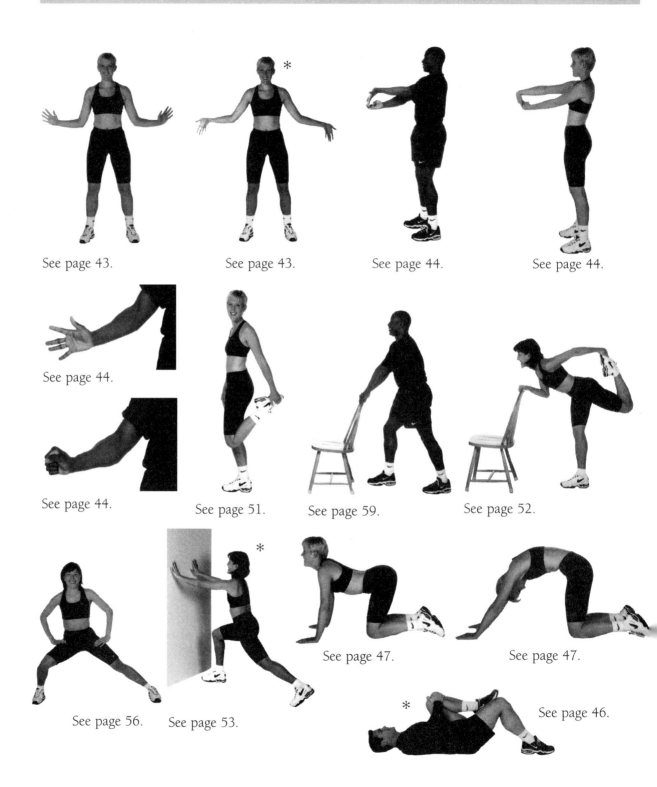

See page 43.

See page 43.

See page 44.

See page 44.

See page 44.

See page 44.

See page 51.

See page 59.

See page 52.

See page 56.

See page 53.

See page 47.

See page 47.

See page 46.

Cross-Country Skiing

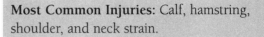

Most Common Injuries: Calf, hamstring, shoulder, and neck strain.

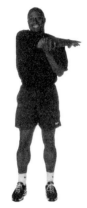

See page 35.

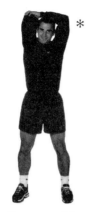

*

See page 36.

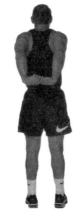

See page 40.

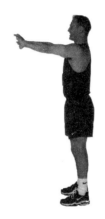

See page 34.

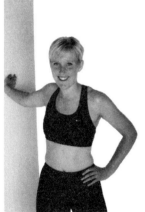

See page 38.

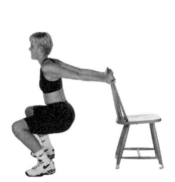

See page 39.

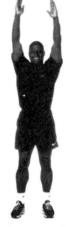

See page 37.

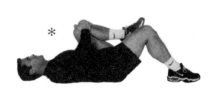

*

See page 46.

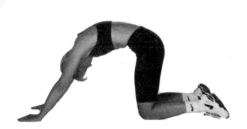

See page 47.

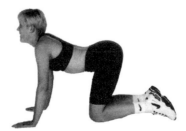

See page 47.

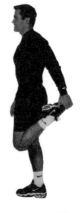

See page 51.

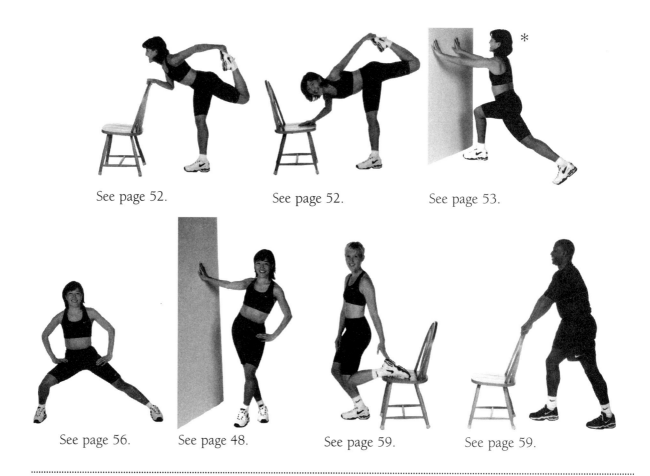

See page 52.　　　　See page 52.　　　　See page 53.

See page 56.　　See page 48.　　See page 59.　　See page 59.

Cycling/Mountain Biking

Cyclists are prone to equipment-related injuries. A hard, non-padded seat can put pressure on the nerve at the base of the buttocks, which can cause temporary impotence in men. Persistent pressure is the major source of nerve injury in the neck and pelvis. Constant leaning on the hands can put pressure on the wrist nerve.

Most Common Injuries: Toe and ankle fracture; hip strain; buttock spasm; neck, shoulder, and forearm muscle strain; nerve damage/compression in the hand and forearm.

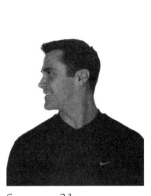
See page 31.

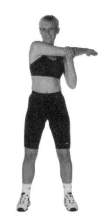 *
See page 33.

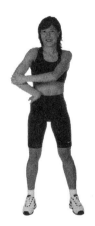
See page 35.

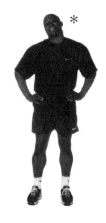
See page 36.

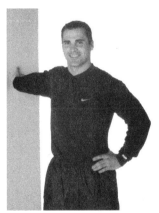
See page 38.

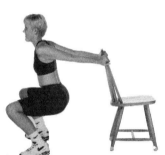
See page 39.

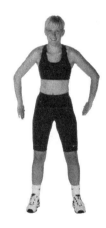
See page 39.

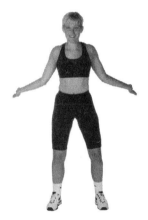
See page 35.

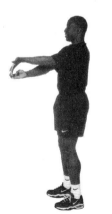
See page 44.

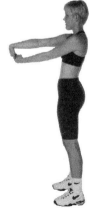
See page 44.

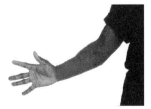
See page 44.

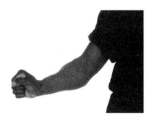
See page 44.

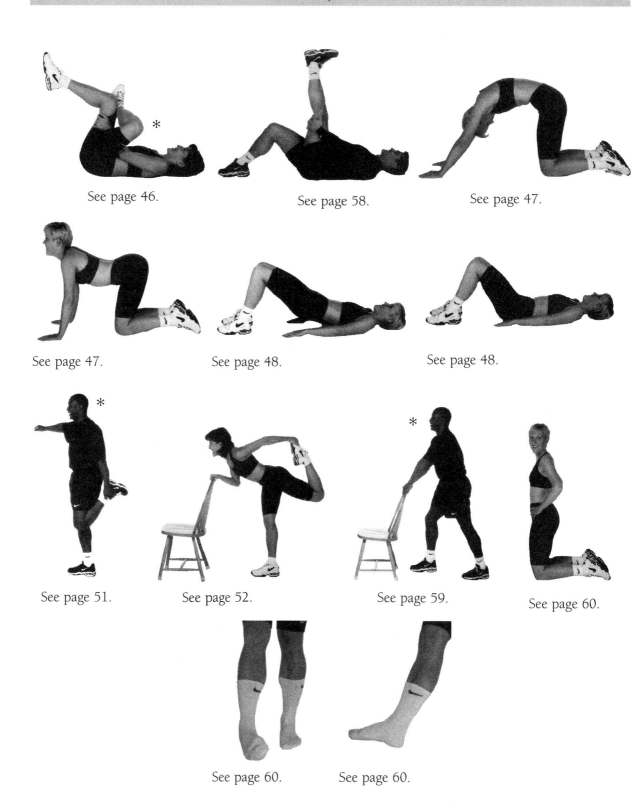

See page 46.

See page 58.

See page 47.

See page 47.

See page 48.

See page 48.

See page 51.

See page 52.

See page 59.

See page 60.

See page 60.

See page 60.

Equestrian (Riding)

Most Common Injuries: Low back, neck, and wrist strain; pelvic fracture; wrist sprain/fracture.

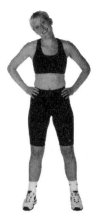

See page 32.

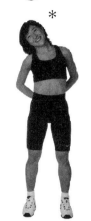
*

See page 32.

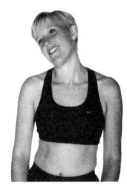

See page 31.

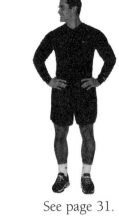

See page 33.

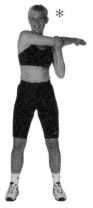
*

See page 35.

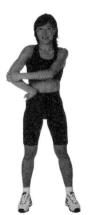

See page 36.

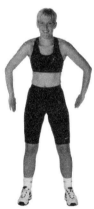

See page 35.

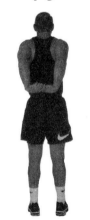

See page 40.

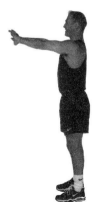

See page 34.

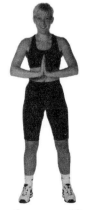

See page 42.

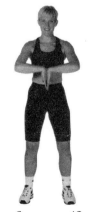

See page 42.

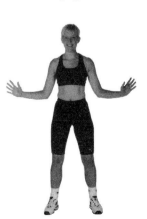

See page 43.

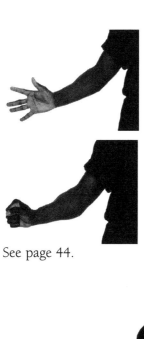

See page 44.

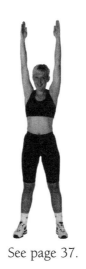

See page 37.

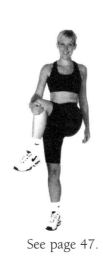

See page 47.

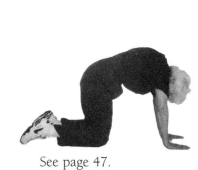

See page 47.

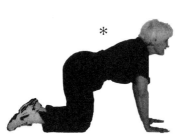

*

See page 47.

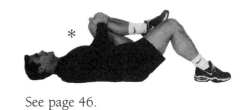

*

See page 46.

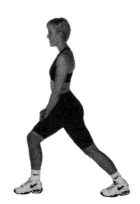

See page 59.

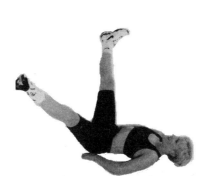

See page 57.

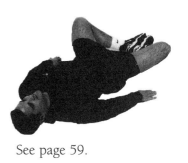

See page 59.

Football/Rugby

In football and rugby, the nerves at the base of the neck, called the brachial plexus, are often damaged because of excessive traction of the arm away from the body and lateral bending of the neck away from the affected side. This is commonly called a "burner" or "stinger." It is usually temporary and causes a sudden pain or weakness down the arm. Many football/rugby players use corticosteroid injections to reduce pain and continue playing when hurt. Corticosteroids weaken collagen, which is the building blocks of muscle tissue. If you hurt, you should rest.

Most Common Injuries: Ankle sprain; knee ligament strain/sprain (medial collateral); low back strain; neck strain/sprain; shoulder and elbow dislocation.

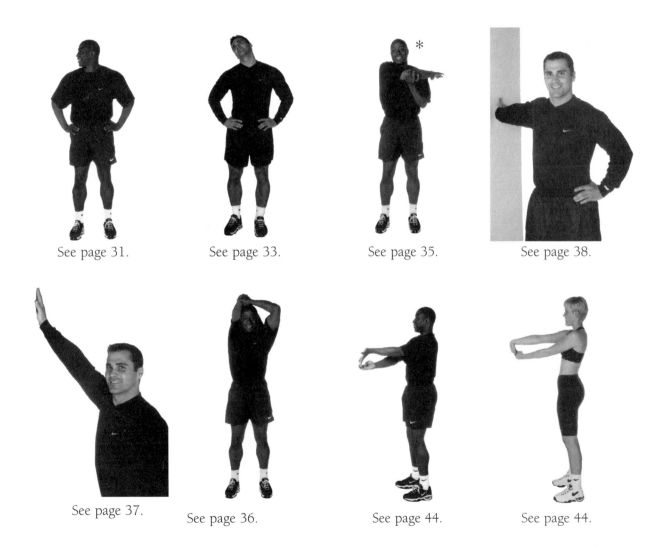

See page 31.   See page 33.   See page 35.   See page 38.

See page 37.   See page 36.   See page 44.   See page 44.

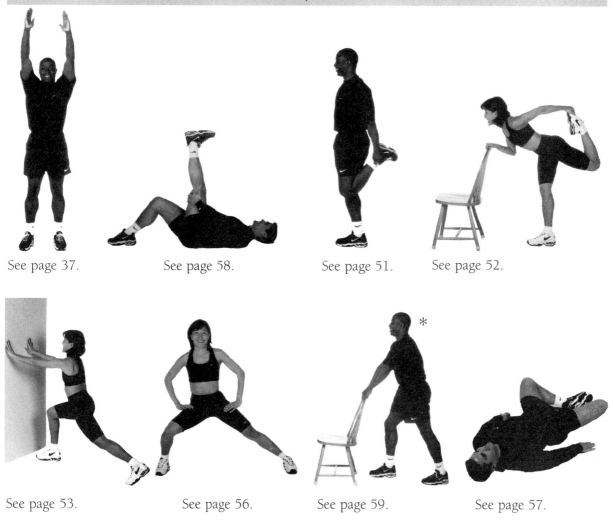

See page 37.　　　See page 58.　　　See page 51.　　See page 52.

See page 53.　　　See page 56.　　　See page 59.　　　See page 57.

Golf

Even though golf is seen by most people as an easy sport, injuries commonly occur. This is due in part to poor technique, which causes spinal joint compression and spinal disc tear.

Most Common Injuries: Low back strain/sprain; herniated disc; shoulder strain; elbow sprain. Golfer's elbow is a strain at the wrist flexor muscles as they attach to the bone at the elbow.

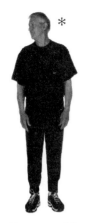

See page 31.

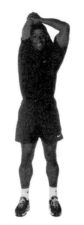

See page 35.

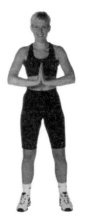

See page 36.

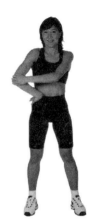

See page 36.

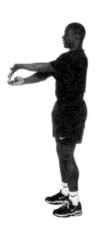

See page 44.

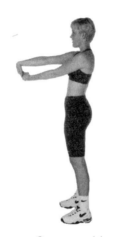

See page 44.

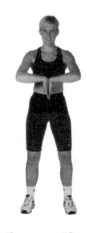

See page 42.

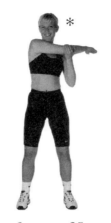

See page 42.

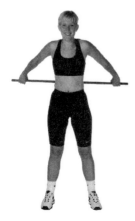

See page 40.

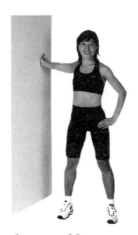

See page 38.

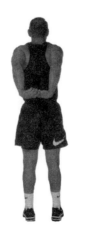

See page 40.

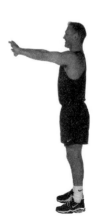

See page 34.

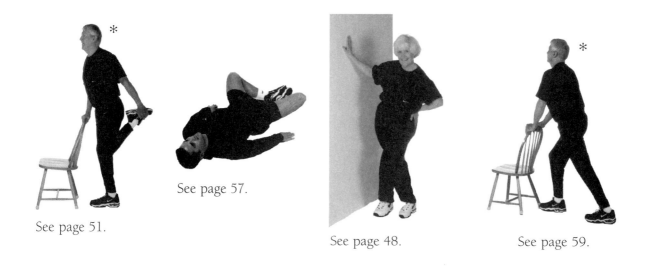

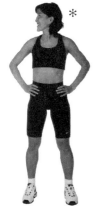

See page 51.

See page 57.

See page 48.

See page 59.

Gymnastics

Gymnasts often impact their hands and elbows when they fall, which can lead to carpal tunnel syndrome—a condition often seen in typists. They can also suffer from severe hyperextension of the body at the waist as well as leg pain and numbness from damage to the femoral nerve, which runs along the front of the thigh.

Most Common Injuries: Spinal joint sprain; back muscle strain; shoulder dislocation; ankle sprain.

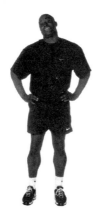

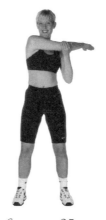

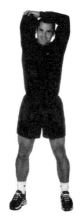

See page 31.

See page 33.

See page 35.

See page 36.

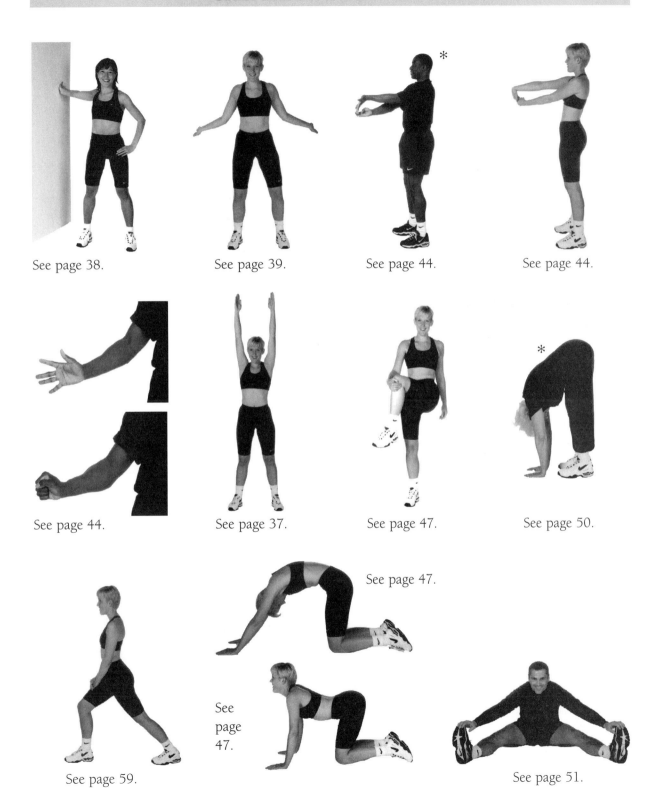

See page 38.

See page 39.

See page 44.

See page 44.

See page 44.

See page 37.

See page 47.

See page 50.

See page 47.

See page 47.

See page 59.

See page 51.

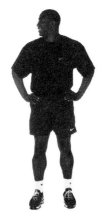

See page 52.

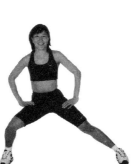

See page 56.

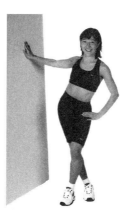

See page 48.

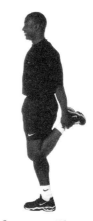

See page 51.

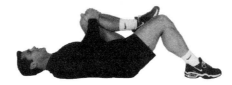

See page 46.

Hockey (Ice and Field)/Lacrosse

Most Common Injuries: Tailbone and clavicle (collarbone) fracture; separation of shoulder joint; neck and low back strain; chest and groin strain; ankle sprain.

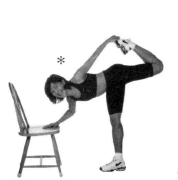

See page 31.

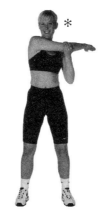

See page 35.

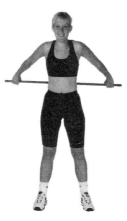

See page 40.

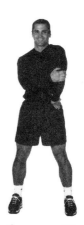

See page 36.

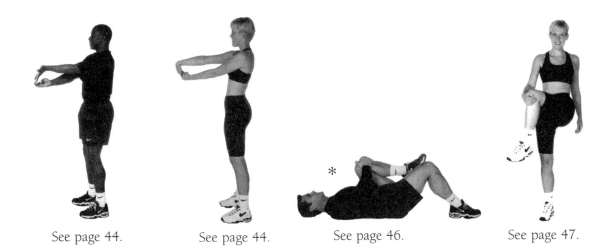

See page 44.   See page 44.   See page 46.   See page 47.

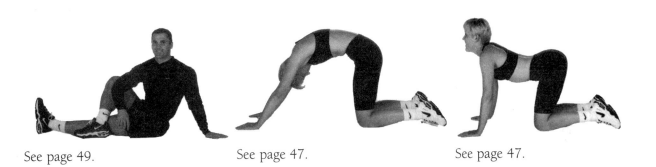

See page 49.   See page 47.   See page 47.

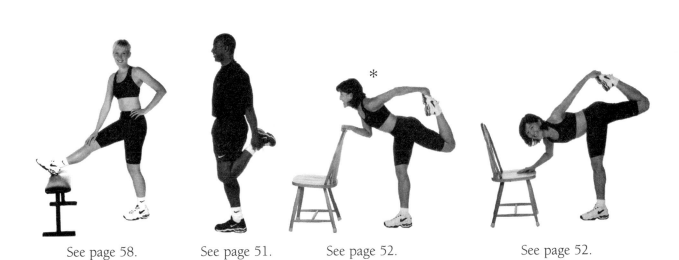

See page 58.   See page 51.   See page 52.   See page 52.

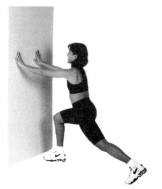

See page 53.

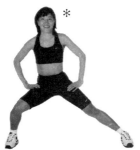

*

See page 56.

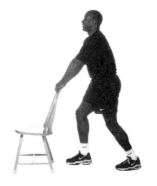

See page 61.

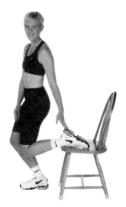

See page 59.

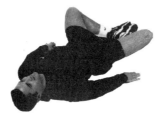

See page 57.

Martial Arts

Most Common Injuries: Neck strain; shoulder dislocation; wrist and finger sprain; back, groin, calf, and hamstring strain; back strain/sprain.

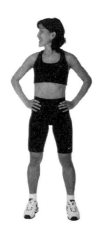

See page 31.

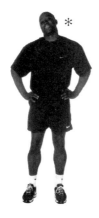

*

See page 33.

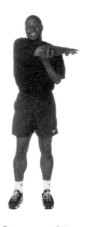

See page 35.

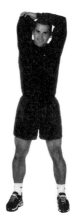

See page 36.

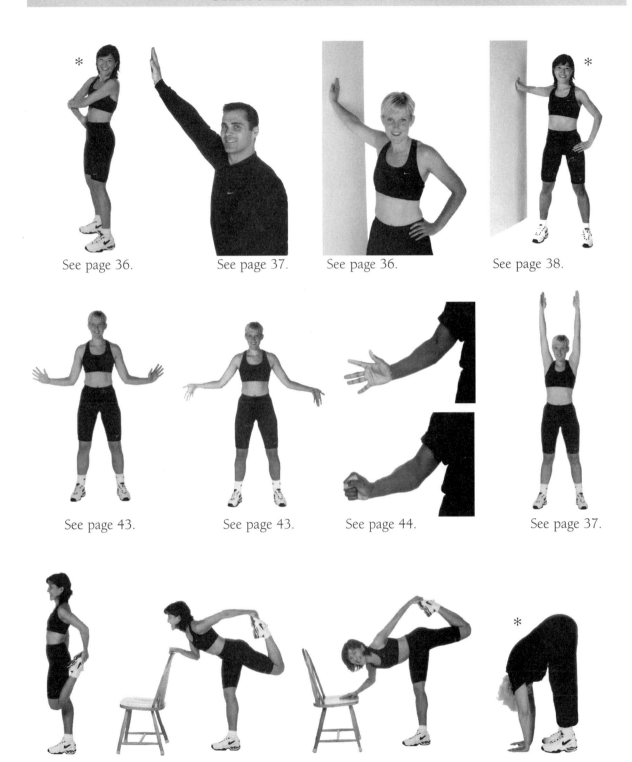

See page 36.　　　See page 37.　　　See page 36.　　　See page 38.

See page 43.　　　See page 43.　　　See page 44.　　　See page 37.

See page 51.　　　See page 52.　　　See page 52.　　　See page 50.

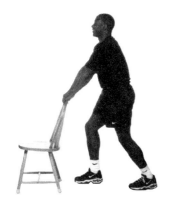

See page 61.

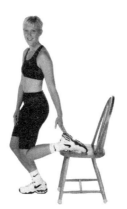

See page 59.

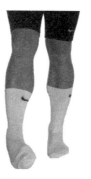

See page 60.

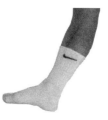

See page 60.

See page 46.

See page 47.

See page 47.

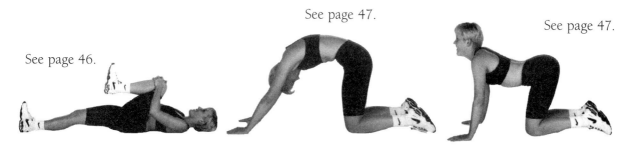

Rowing

Most Common Injuries: Hamstring, low back, neck, and shoulder strain.

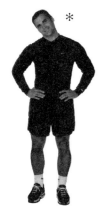

See page 32.

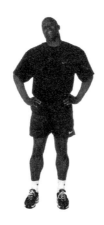

See page 33.

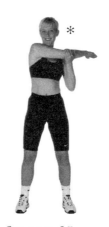

See page 35.

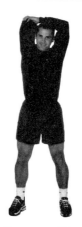

See page 36.

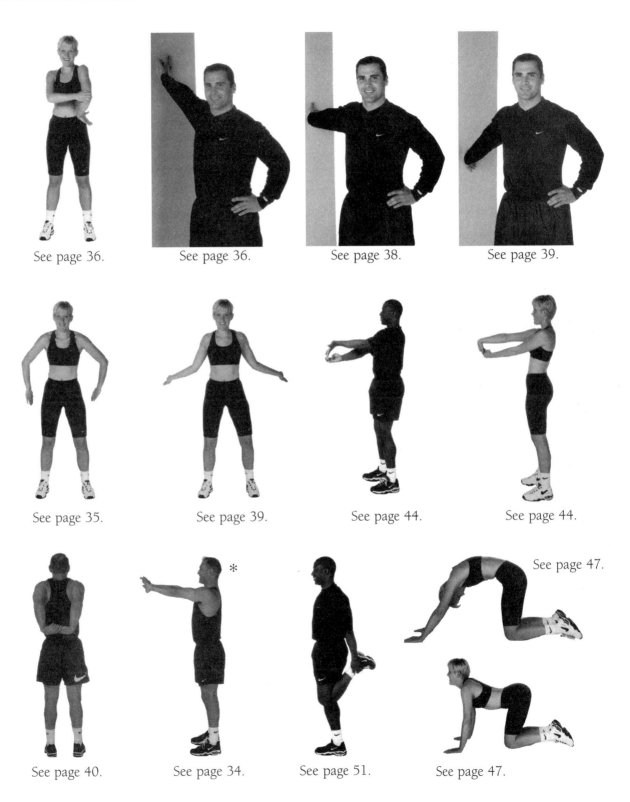

See page 36.

See page 36.

See page 38.

See page 39.

See page 35.

See page 39.

See page 44.

See page 44.

See page 47.

*

See page 40.

See page 34.

See page 51.

See page 47.

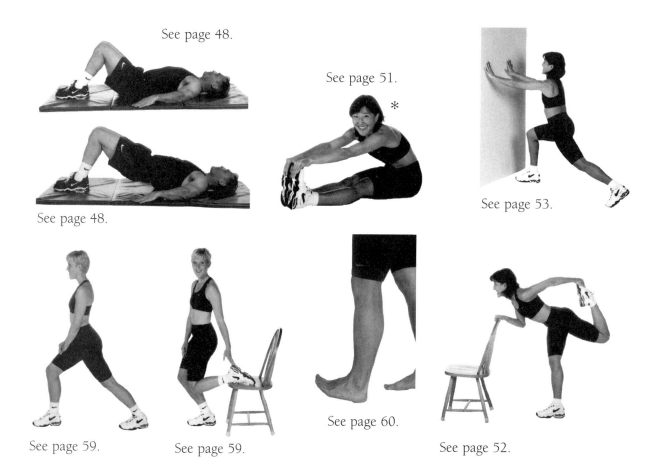

See page 48.

See page 48.

See page 51.

See page 53.

See page 59.

See page 59.

See page 60.

See page 52.

Running/Walking

Running can generate up to six times the force of a person's body weight through the body. Up to 15% of runners suffer from nerve damage, which is experienced as chronic foot pain. They may also experience sciatica, which is pain that runs from the low back down the leg to the toe. Sciatica can occur from low back disc rupture, spasm of the buttock muscle, or compression in the back of the knee region. Walking, on the other hand, rarely causes nerve damage. If you do speed walking, however, make sure that you have a good technique; otherwise, you can develop neck, back, knee, foot, and ankle injuries.

Most Common Injuries: Achilles tendon, hip, and low back strain; calf spasm; neck and shoulder stiffness.

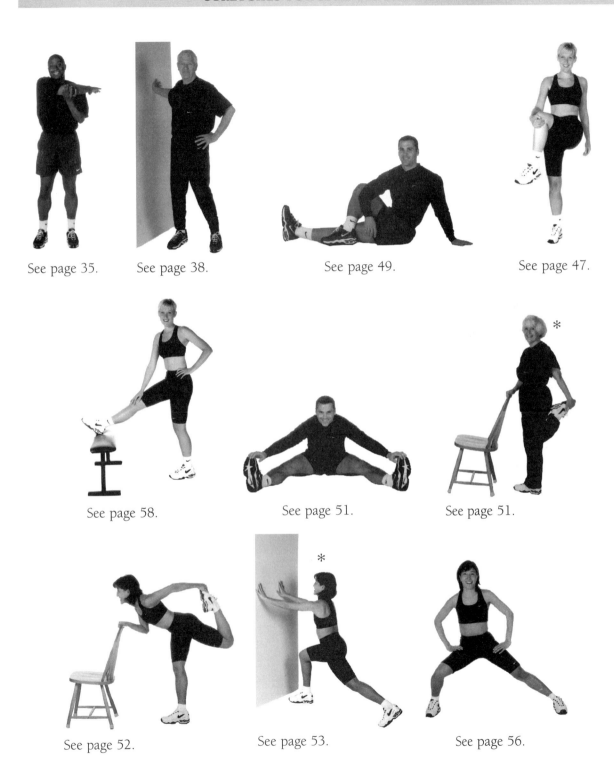

See page 35.   See page 38.   See page 49.   See page 47.

See page 58.   See page 51.   See page 51.

See page 52.   See page 53.   See page 56.

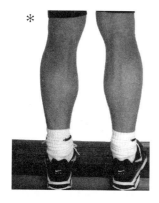

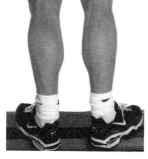

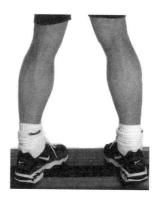

* See page 61.   See page 61.   See page 61.

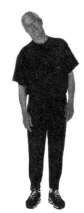

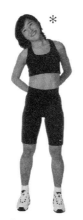

* See page 59.

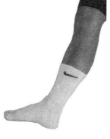

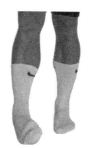

See page 60.   See page 60.

Sailing

Most Common Injuries: Neck joint jamming; strain in front of shoulder; frozen shoulder; wrist and low back strain; lumbar disc herniation.

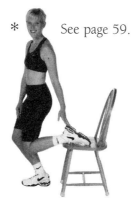

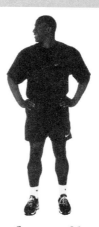

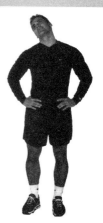

See page 32.   See page 32.   See page 31.   See page 33.

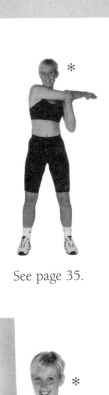 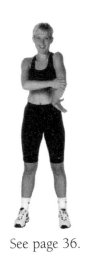 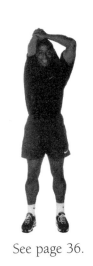 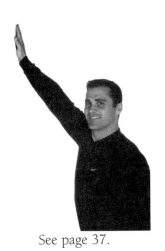

See page 35.   See page 36.   See page 36.   See page 37.

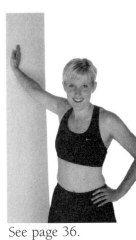 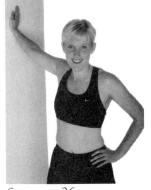 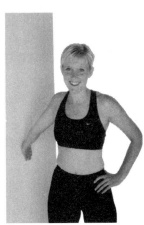 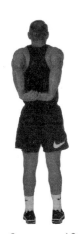

See page 38.   See page 36.   See page 39.   See page 40.

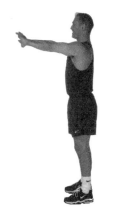 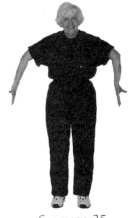 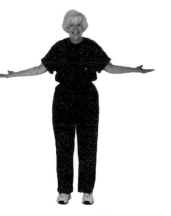 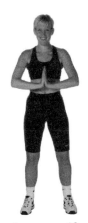

See page 34.   See page 35.   See page 39.   See page 42.

111

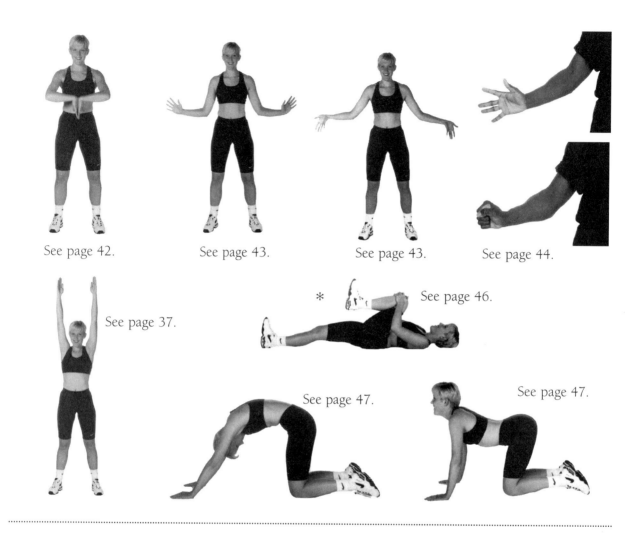

See page 42.

See page 43.

See page 43.

See page 44.

See page 37.

* See page 46.

See page 47.

See page 47.

Skating

Most Common Injuries: Groin and low back strain; tailbone fracture; wrist hyperextension/strain; sciatica.

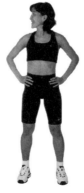

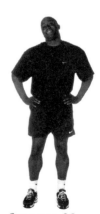

See page 31.

See page 33.

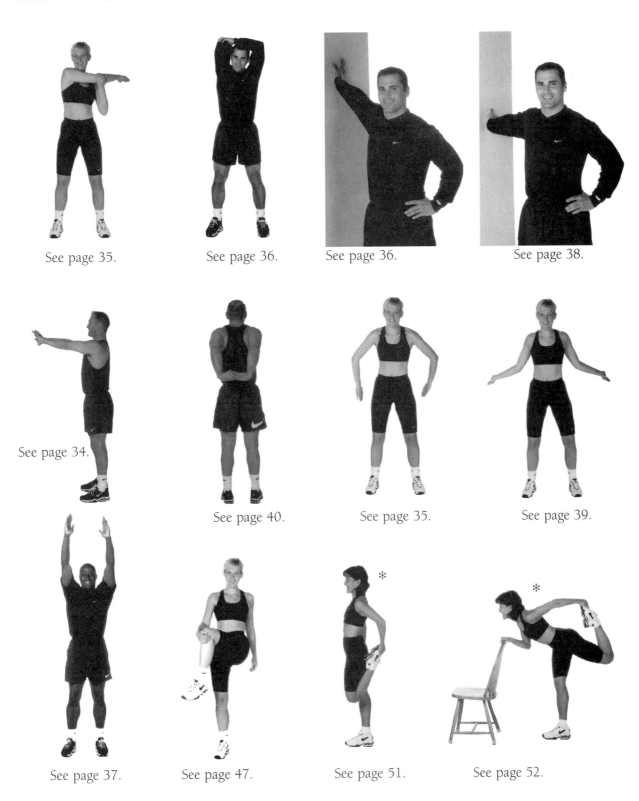

See page 35.

See page 36.

See page 36.

See page 38.

See page 34.

See page 40.

See page 35.

See page 39.

See page 37.

See page 47.

See page 51.

See page 52.

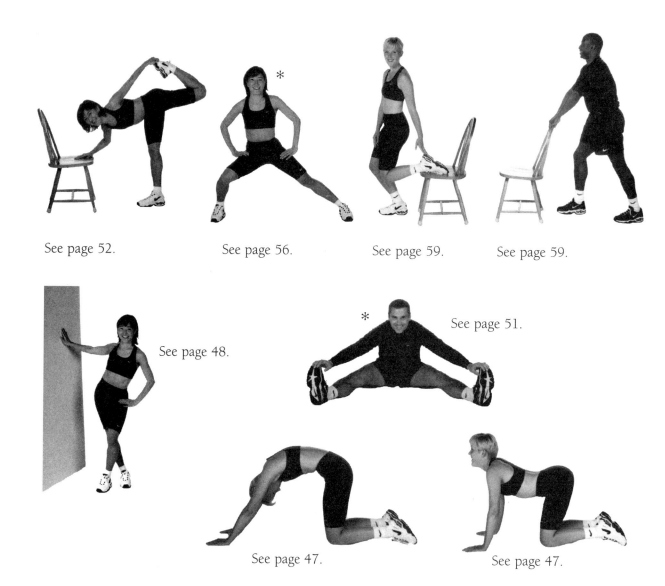

See page 52.

See page 56.

See page 59.

See page 59.

See page 48.

See page 51.

See page 47.

See page 47.

Soccer

Most Common Injuries: Achilles strain/tear; hamstring strain; knee and low back strain/sprain.

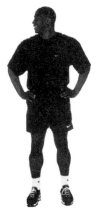

See page 31.

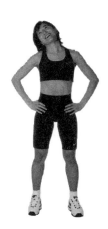

See page 33.

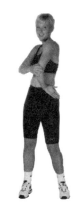

See page 36.

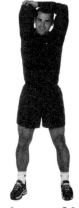

See page 36.

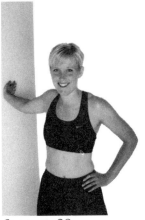

See page 38.

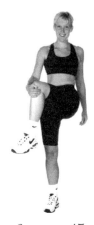

See page 47.

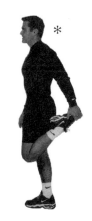

See page 51.

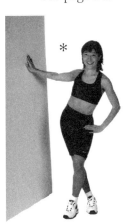

See page 48.

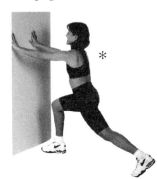

See page 53.

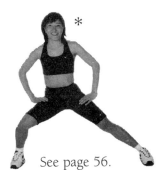

See page 56.

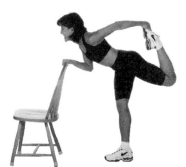

See page 52.

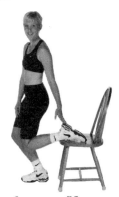

See page 59.

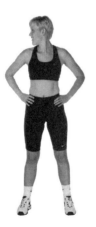 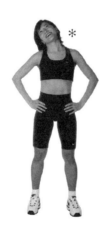 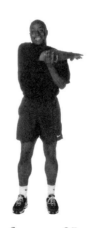 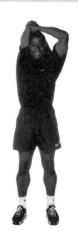

| See page 59. | See page 61. | See page 51. | See page 57. |

Squash/Racquetball/ Tennis

Most Common Injuries: Achilles tendon, groin, low back, elbow, and wrist strain (tennis elbow); buttocks stiffness; osteoarthritis of the hip (particularly from squash).

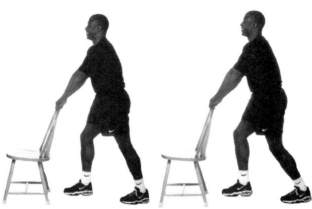 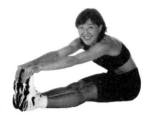 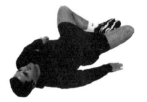

| See page 31. | See page 33. | See page 35. | See page 36. |

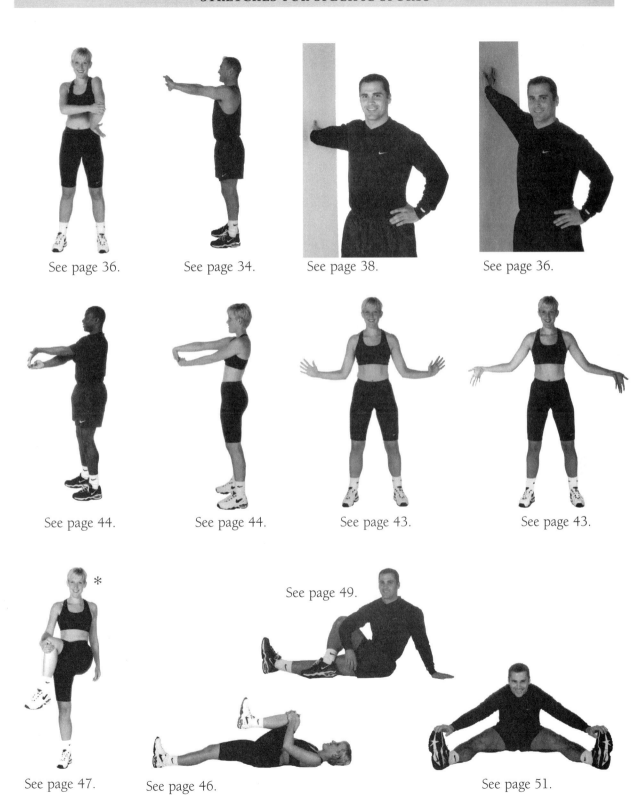

See page 36.

See page 34.

See page 38.

See page 36.

See page 44.

See page 44.

See page 43.

See page 43.

*

See page 49.

See page 47.

See page 46.

See page 51.

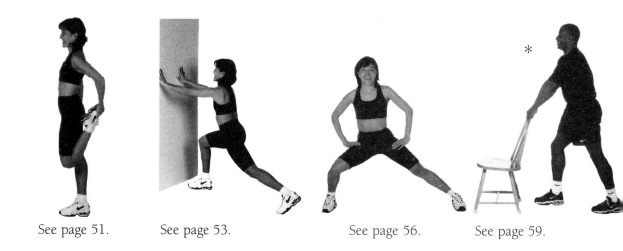

See page 51.   See page 53.   See page 56.   See page 59.

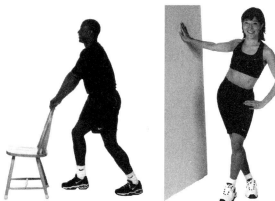

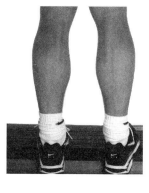

See page 61.   See page 48.

See page 61.

Snowboarding/ Kneeboarding

Most Common Injuries: 1) Snowboarding: Shoulder separation/dislocation; rib strain/fracture; neck, chest, and low back strain; wrist sprain; wrist and thumb fracture.
2) Kneeboarding: Neck hyperflexion and extension; shoulder dislocation; knee hyperflexion; ankle hyperextension; strains.

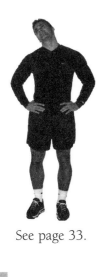

See page 33.

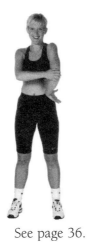

See page 36.

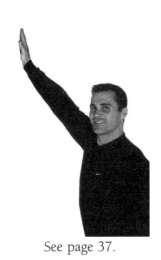

See page 37.

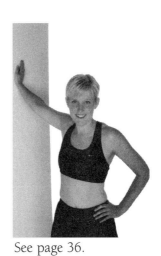

See page 36.

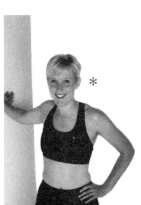

See page 38.

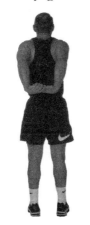

See page 40.

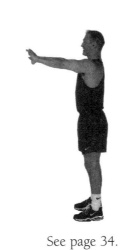

See page 34.

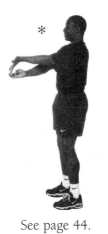

See page 44.

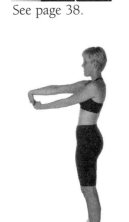

See page 44.

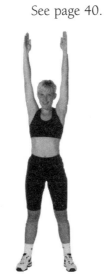

See page 37.

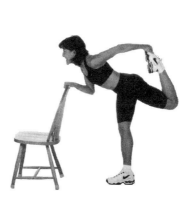

See page 52.

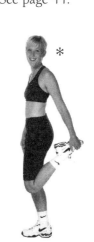

See page 51.

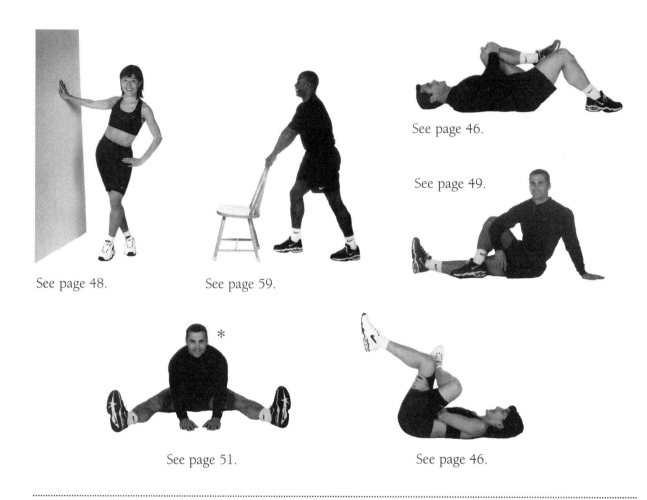

See page 48.

See page 59.

See page 46.

See page 49.

See page 51.

See page 46.

Swimming

Swimming, like walking, does not cause any nerve damage. The water counteracts the effects of gravity. Swimming both stretches and strengthens the entire body. It is our favorite exercise, as it offers significant reward at very little risk. However, if you do a great deal of front crawl, you should learn to breathe on both sides to avoid neck muscle/joint and nerve irritation.

Most Common Injuries: Shoulder (rotator cuff) strain; neck stiffness; neck nerve irritation.

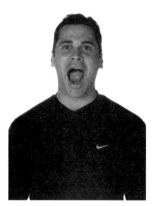

See page 29.

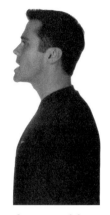

See page 29.

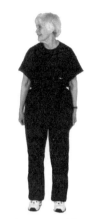

See page 32.

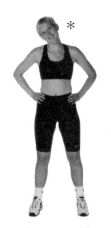

See page 31.

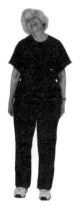

See page 33.

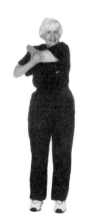

See page 35.

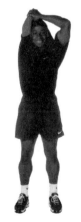

See page 36.

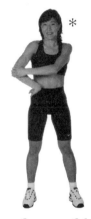

See page 36.

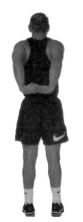

See page 40.

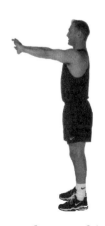

See page 34.

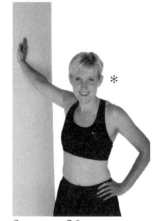

See page 36.

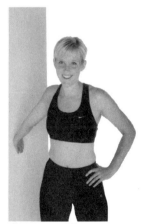

See page 39.

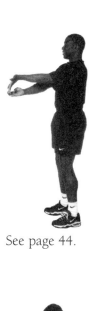

See page 44.

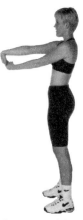

See page 44.

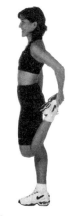

See page 51.

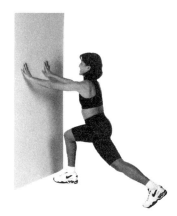

See page 53.

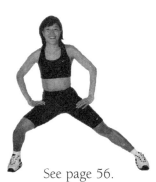

See page 56.

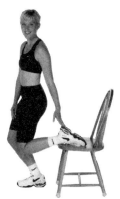

See page 59.

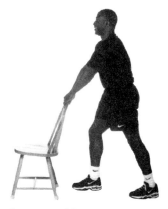

See page 59.

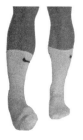

See page 60.

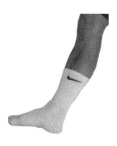

See page 60.

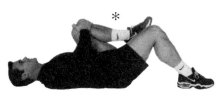

*

See page 46.

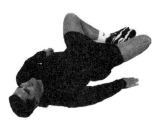

See page 57.

Waterskiing

Most Common Injuries: Shoulder strain/separation; biceps, forearm, neck, and back strain; hamstring pull.

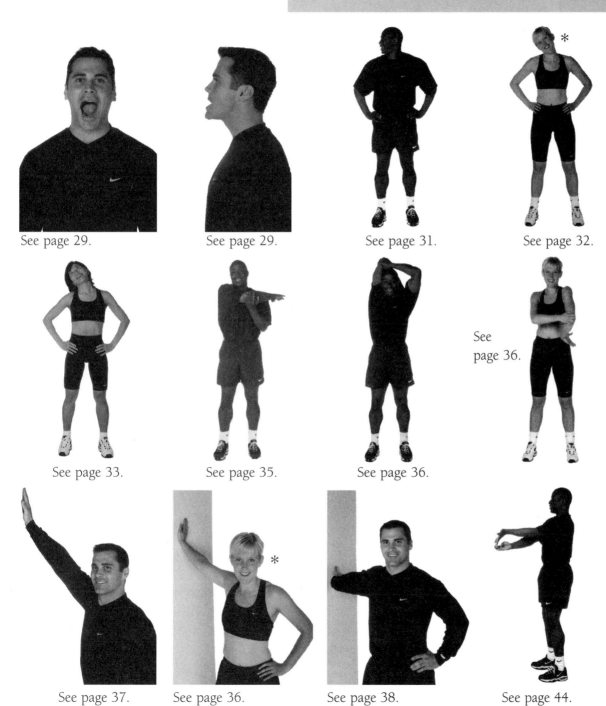

See page 29.

See page 29.

See page 31.

See page 32. *

See page 33.

See page 35.

See page 36.

See page 36.

See page 37.

See page 36. *

See page 38.

See page 44.

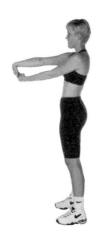 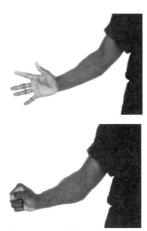 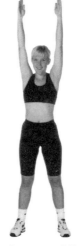 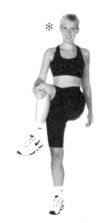

See page 44. See page 44. See page 37. See page 47.

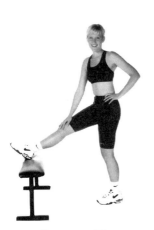 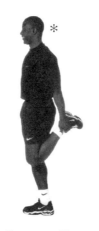 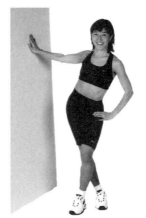 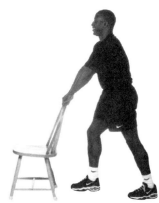

See page 58. See page 51. See page 48. See page 59.

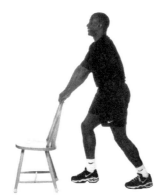 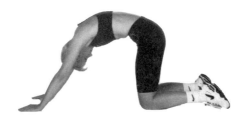 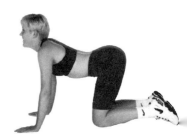

See page 47. See page 47.

See page 61.

Weight Lifting/ Bodybuilding

Most Common Injuries: *Squats:* Low back strain; sciatica; herniated disc; knee ligament damage. *Shoulder press:* Shoulder tendonitis; upper rib misalignment. *Upright row:* Front neck/nerve traction causing tingling/pain down arms. *Bench press:* Rib and upper back strain. *Bent-over row:* Low back ligament strain. *Dead lifts:* Low back ligament strain; disc injury.

We suggest that you stretch the muscle just exercised for 30 seconds between sets. Then redo these stretches during the cool-down.

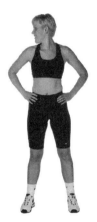

See page 31.

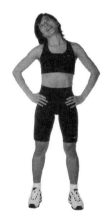

See page 33.

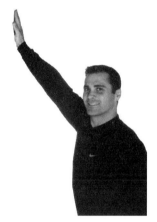

See page 37.

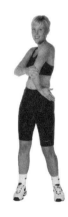

See page 36.

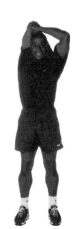

See page 36.

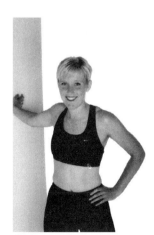

See page 38.

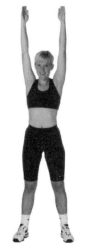

See page 37.

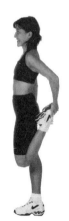

See page 51.

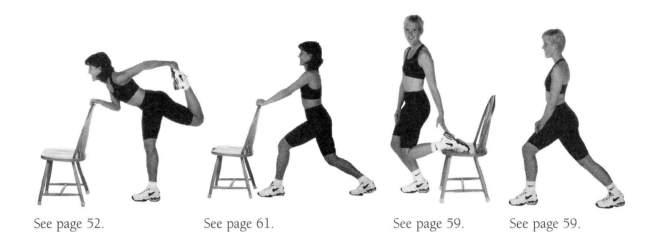

See page 52. See page 61. See page 59. See page 59.

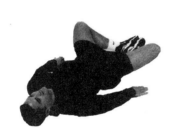

See page 57.

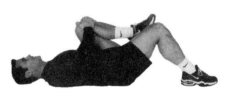

See page 46.

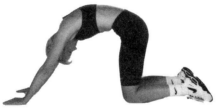

See page 47.

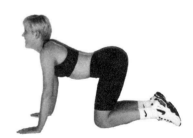

See page 47.

Stretching for Injury Rehabilitation & Pain Syndromes

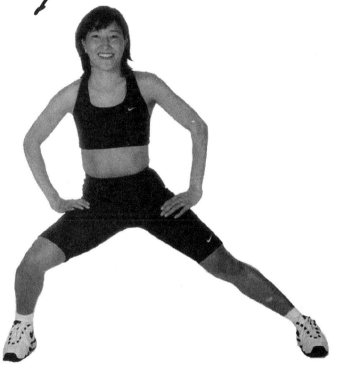

*P*ain can arise in virtually any tissue in the body. But it would take several volumes just to understand all of the concepts and recent theories regarding various pain symptoms. However, if you have a good understanding of the basic concept of pain (see Chapter 5) and anatomy (see Chapter 7), you will be better able to deal with and manage many disorders that may arise.

The following nineteen disorders or conditions are the most common problems that people have experienced at some time. The specific stretches for each condition will help reduce pain frequency, intensity, and duration. But always remember that if the pain persists, consult your physician and chiropractor. If you have already been diagnosed with any one of the following syndromes, you should talk with your physician about incorporating the relevant stretches into a regular flexibility program. It can optimize your health and quicken your recovery.

Achilles Tendonitis/ Calf Strain

Prolonged wearing of high heel shoes can lead to chronic shortening of the calf and Achilles tendon, which leads to injury. Achilles tendonitis generally occurs from overuse with insufficient stretching. Calf strain usually occurs from underuse with inadequate stretching prior to exercise. Both conditions can be managed in a similar way.

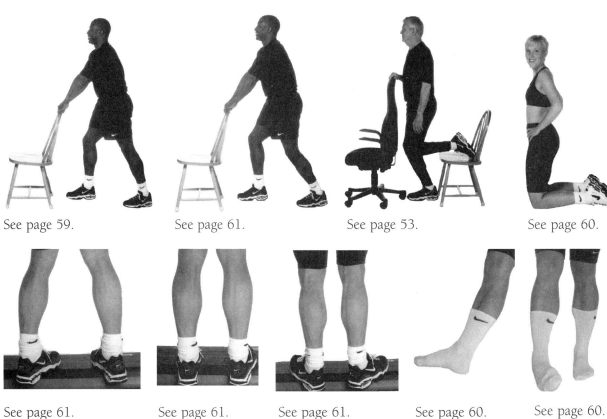

See page 59.   See page 61.   See page 53.   See page 60.

See page 61.   See page 61.   See page 61.   See page 60.   See page 60.

See page 54.

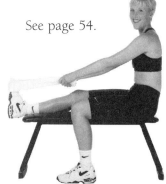

Ankle Sprains

Ankle sprains often result from mechanical imbalances in the muscles and ligaments of the pelvis and lower limbs. There are two types of ankle sprains: eversion and inversion. Eversion sprains are generally referred to as a "going over" or "rolling over" of the ankle. When this happens, the ankle rolls over past its normal limit so that the sole of the foot faces inward towards the other ankle. Most ankle sprains are eversion. An inversion sprain is when the sole of the foot is sprained outwards. This kind of sprain occurs only about 5% of the time. To prevent ankle sprains, stretch and strengthen the ankle joint and associated muscles. Rehabilitation involves rest, elevation, ice, compression in the early phase, and stretching (the muscles on the opposite side of the sprain) and exercise (particularly calf raises) in the later phase.

EVERSION SPRAINS:

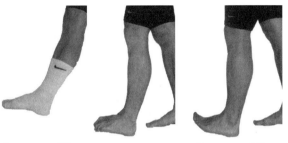

See page 60. See page 60. See page 60.

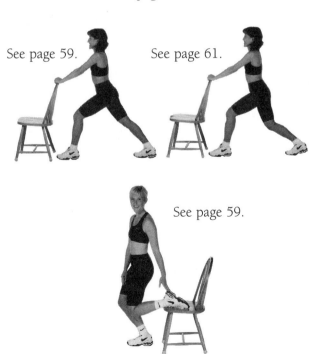

See page 59. See page 61.

See page 59.

INVERSION SPRAINS:

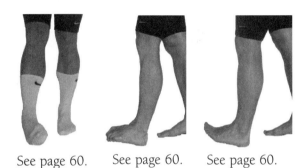

See page 60. See page 60. See page 60.

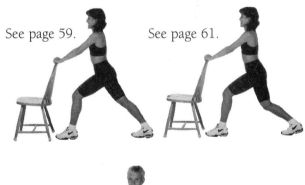

See page 59. See page 61.

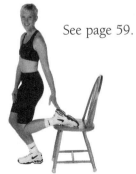

See page 59.

Asthma

Asthma is a chronic, obstructive lung disorder that blocks air travel in the tubes of the lungs to cause a shortness of breath. The restricted breathing pattern that occurs can often lead to a stiffening of the rib cage, neck, and middle back mus-

cles. This can be greatly minimized by the following stretches.

These stretches can also be used by someone who has recovered from chest surgeries and/or rib fractures. Consult your physician about using them as part of rehabilitation to minimize the scar tissue formation in the muscles.

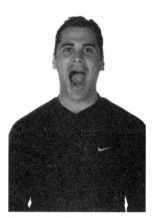
See page 29.

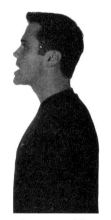
See page 29.

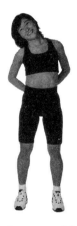
See page 32.

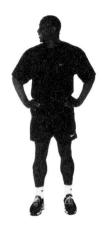
See page 31.

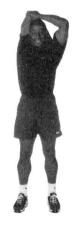
See page 36.

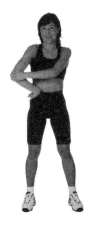
See page 36.

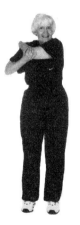
See page 35.

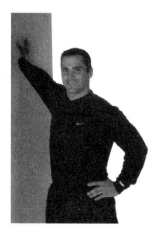
See page 36.

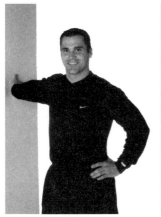

See page 38.

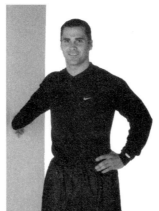

See page 39.

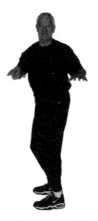

See page 49.

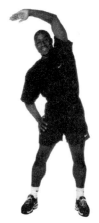

See page 37.

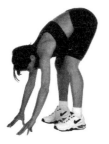

See page 50.

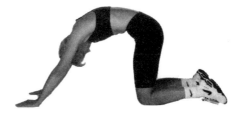

See page 47.

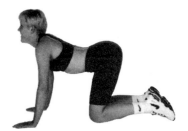

See page 47.

Shoulder Pain

Whether standing or sitting, a person slouching will "round" his or her shoulders forward. Over time, the chest muscles adaptively shorten and the shoulder blade muscles lengthen so that each area will feel sore. The muscles supporting the spine and rib cage will then no longer function optimally. As a result, impaired breathing can occur. To compensate for the irregular stresses placed in these regions, the muscles will then change their structure and mechanics. Since the neck nerves make the shoulder and chest muscles function, neck stretches are necessary.

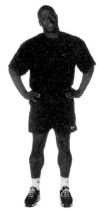
See page 32.

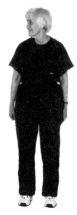
See page 31.

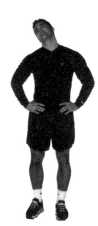
See page 33.

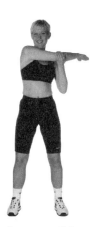
See page 35.

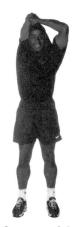
See page 36.

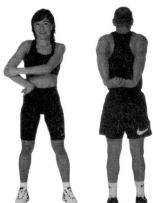
See page 36.   See page 40.

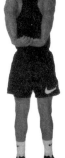

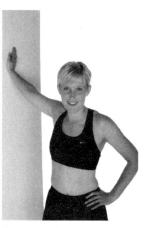
See page 36.

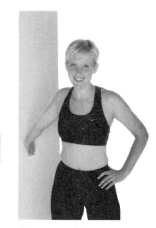
See page 38.

See page 39.

Frozen Shoulder

A frozen shoulder is the result of long-term repetitive irritation and inflammation, and/or degenerative disc disease in the neck. Repetitive strain often causes scar tissues, or adhesions, to accumulate in the ligaments, muscles, and tendons of the shoulder. The increased stiffness reduces the range of motion in the shoulder. Trauma as well as previous neck injuries can cause a frozen shoulder.

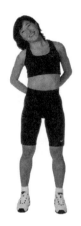

See page 32.

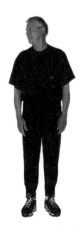

See page 31.

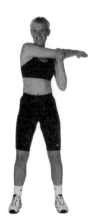

See page 35.

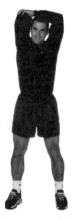

See page 36.

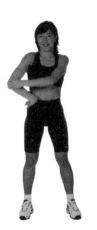

See page 36.

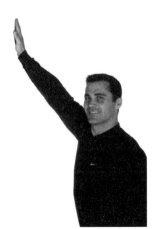

See page 37.

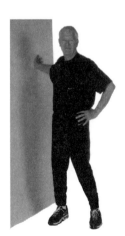

See page 38.

Golfer's Elbow

This condition, which often happens to golfers, occurs from repetitive stress or strain to the elbow region where the tendons attach to the bones (generally on the inside of the elbow when the palm faces forward). People who develop this problem often neglect to do forearm stretches. Doing it will reduce the incidence of this injury, and ice can treat it if it has swollen from overuse. Neck nerve irritation is also one of the causes of forearm muscle dysfunction. Remember, corticosteroid injection may initially reduce swelling, but it weakens the building blocks (collagen) of the muscle in the long run, which makes you more prone to recurrences.

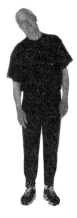

See page 32.

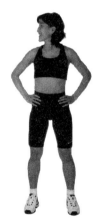

See page 31.

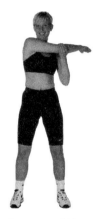

See page 33.

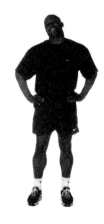

See page 35.

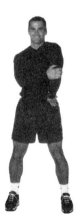

See page 36.

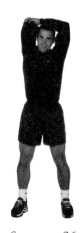

See page 36.

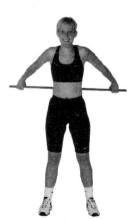

See page 40.

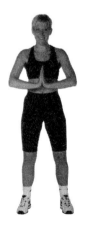

See page 42.

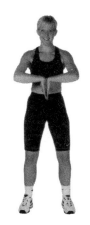

See page 42.

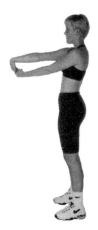
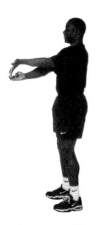

See page 44.

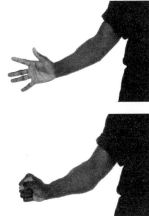

See page 44.

See page 44.

Tennis Elbow

This condition is the opposite of a golfer's elbow. It is caused by repetitive stress to the muscles on the back of the forearm (generally, the outside of the elbow when the palm faces forward). The tighter muscles pull the tendon from where it attaches to the bone and create inflammation. Ice, stretching, and rest are excellent ways to start rehabilitation. Chiropractic care can improve elbow, shoulder, and neck mechanics to promote healing. Recent studies have found that corticosteroid injections should not be used to treat this condition. Weakened muscles and tendon ruptures can happen as a result.

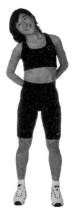

See page 32.

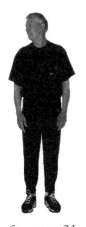

See page 31.

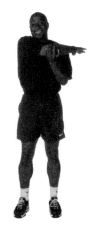

See page 35.

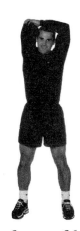

See page 36.

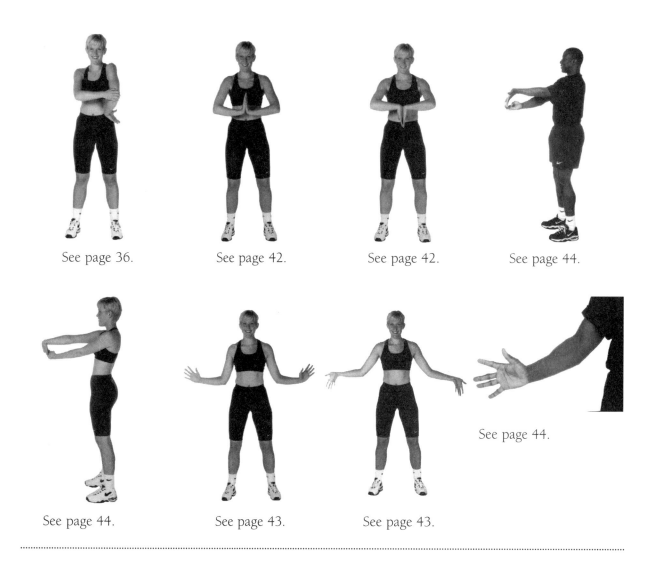

See page 36.

See page 42.

See page 42.

See page 44.

See page 44.

See page 43.

See page 43.

See page 44.

Groin Strain

This injury involves the sudden pulling of the knee outwards from the hip as the result of continuous small traumas (microtraumas) or one sudden trauma. The trauma can come from work, exercise, etc., and, because the low back and/or groin region is too tight, the muscle cannot adapt. Stretching helps the healing process by keeping the region mobile. Be *very gentle* when you begin the stretches.

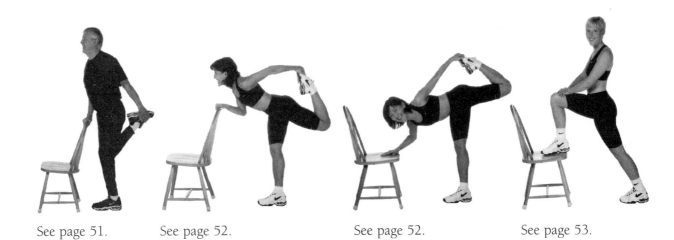

See page 51.   See page 52.   See page 52.   See page 53.

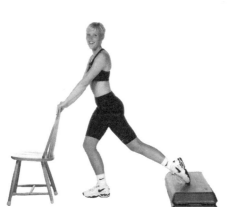

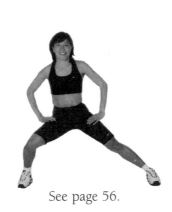

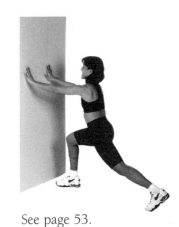

See page 53.

See page 56.

See page 53.

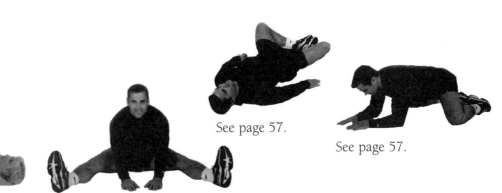

See page 57.

See page 57.

See page 57.   See page 51.

Hip Bursitis

The bursa is a sac of fluid at the top of the thigh bone (femur). The hip bursa prevents the thigh muscles from wearing on the hip bone beneath it. Insufficient leg muscle stretching prior to exercise creates an unexpected pressure on the tendon and consequently the bursa. The pain is often so intense that it can wake you up from sleep. Pain can radiate down the leg and into the shin in severe cases.

More cases of hip bursitis exist today because of step aerobics and stairclimbing exercise equipment. These exercises should be alternated with cycling, swimming, walking, and so on, especially if problems in the hip region are developing. Stretching and manipulation are the best ways to restore normal joint function.

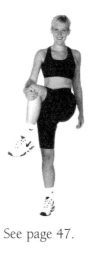

See page 47.

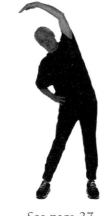

See page 37.

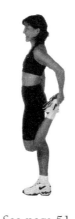

See page 51.

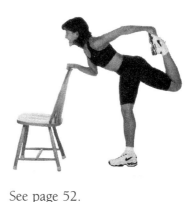

See page 52.

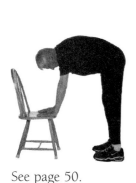

See page 50.

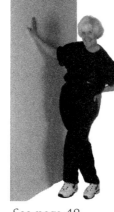

See page 48.

See page 49.

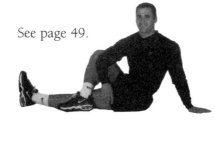

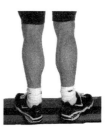

See page 61.

See page 46.

Knee Bursitis

Similar to the hip, the knee also has a bursa. It is located in the front, upper, and inner portion of the shin at the tibia bone. The bursa prevents the tendons from wearing on the knee joint where the hamstrings, thigh, and groin muscles unite. In our experience, the most common cause of knee bursitis is low back and pelvic dysfunction. Ice and stretching are an excellent start toward healing.

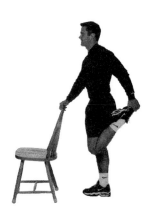

See page 51.

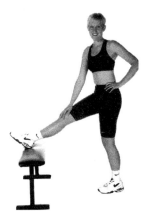

See page 58.

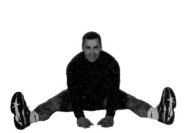

See page 51.

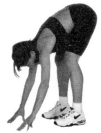

See page 50.

Patellofemoral Disorder

This is a condition where the knee cap (which is rounded on the top and V-shaped on the bottom) does not smoothly move through its groove formed by the thigh bone (femur) beneath it. Traditionally, it has been seen as the result of a weakness in the inner thigh muscle or an overdevelopment of the outer thigh muscle. Quite often it is caused by a pelvic imbalance, an anatomical short leg, abnormal foot/ankle mechanics, lumbar nerve root irritation, improper training, or lack of mobility.

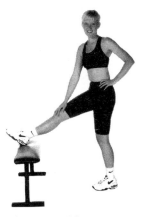

See page 58.

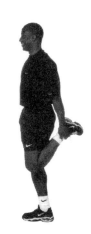

See page 51.

139

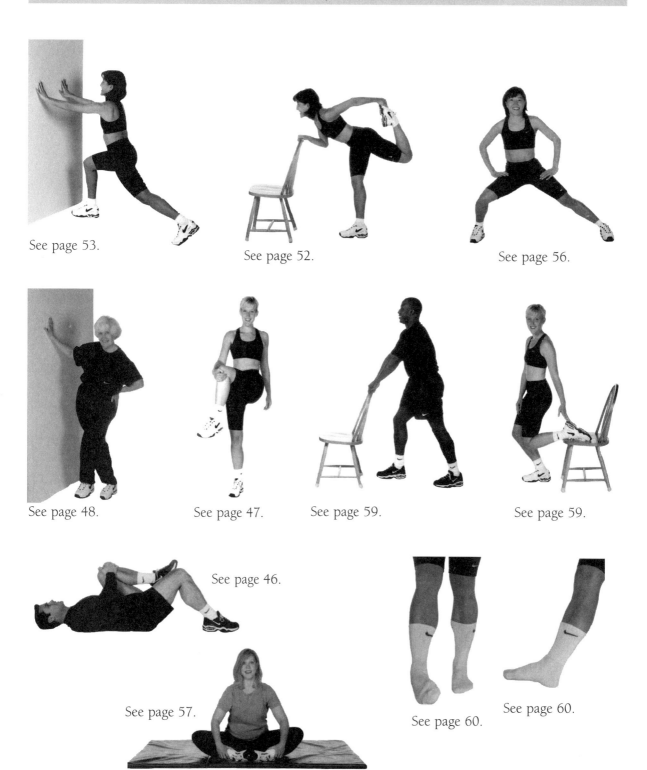

See page 53.

See page 52.

See page 56.

See page 48.

See page 47.

See page 59.

See page 59.

See page 46.

See page 57.

See page 60.

See page 60.

Low Back

Up to 80% of the population experience low back pain at some time in their life. Next to the common cold, low back pain is the most common reason for doctor visits. Its causes are endless. However, at least 80% of cases result from mechanical dysfunction of the back muscles and joints. Stretching must include the legs, pelvis, and back. Although pain medication (acetaminophen, ibuprofen, and aspirin) may help alleviate back pain, you should not use them long term. Scientific research indicates that 85% of musculoskeletal problems recur. Unless properly treated, once you have a weakness, it will always be a weakness. Your chiropractor is the best person to diagnose and treat low back problems.

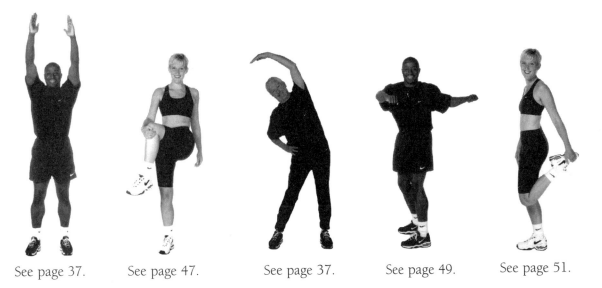

See page 37.   See page 47.   See page 37.   See page 49.   See page 51.

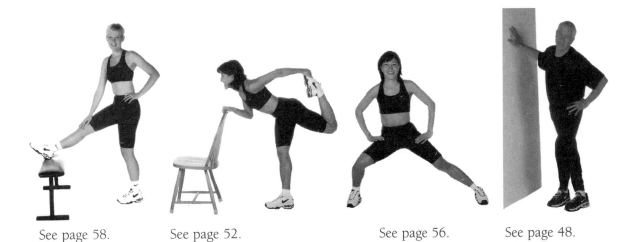

See page 58.   See page 52.   See page 56.   See page 48.

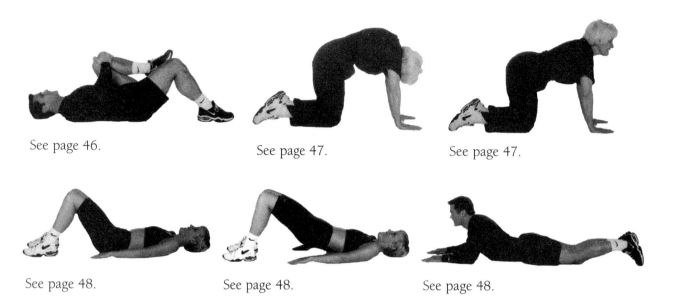

See page 46.   See page 47.   See page 47.

See page 48.   See page 48.   See page 48.

Sciatica

Most people do not suffer from sciatica. Instead, they experience referred pain from the low back into the legs. True sciatica is quite rare. It is the result of pinching of the large sciatic nerve, which is the congregation of the lumbar and sacral spinal nerves. The sciatic nerve runs down the back of the thigh into the leg and foot. The lumbar bones and surrounding soft tissue com-press the nerve to cause the "classic" sciatic pain. The pain can be felt in any of the regions where the nerve travels. It feels like an electrical shock down the legs. See your chiropractor to see if you have true sciatica. If you do, we suggest you use *extreme caution* when stretching, as it may aggravate your condition if done at the wrong time or too quickly. You can always begin with the stretches that provide relief and ignore the ones that aggravate your condition.

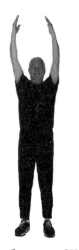

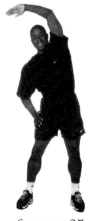

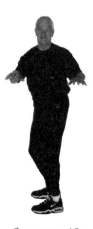

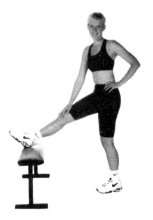

See page 37.

                See page 37.   See page 49.   See page 58.

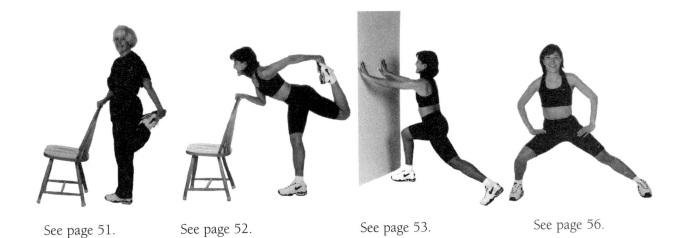

See page 51.　　　See page 52.　　　See page 53.　　　See page 56.

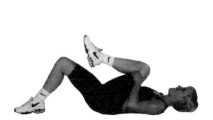

See page 46.　　　See page 46.

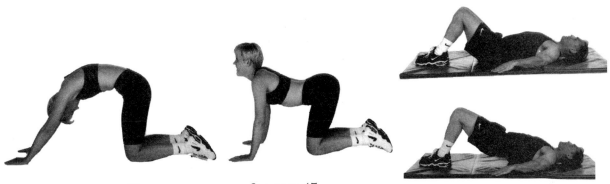

See page 47.　　　See page 47.

See page 48.

Piriformis Syndrome

The piriformis muscle is a small muscle deep in the buttocks region that helps the femur (thigh bone) rotate the thigh outwards (external rotation). The sciatic nerve travels just under (or through) this muscle. Any mild shortening of the piriformis can result in nerve irritation and refer pain to the buttocks, hamstrings, calf, and/or foot. As a result, it is often confused with sciatica. The pelvic joint has a very close relationship to the function of the piriformis. A dysfunctional sacroiliac joint can cause nerve irritation and piriformis shortening. Stretching and ice therapy should quickly reduce this pain syndrome. Begin the stretching very gently. If pain persists for more than 2–4 days, consult your chiropractor.

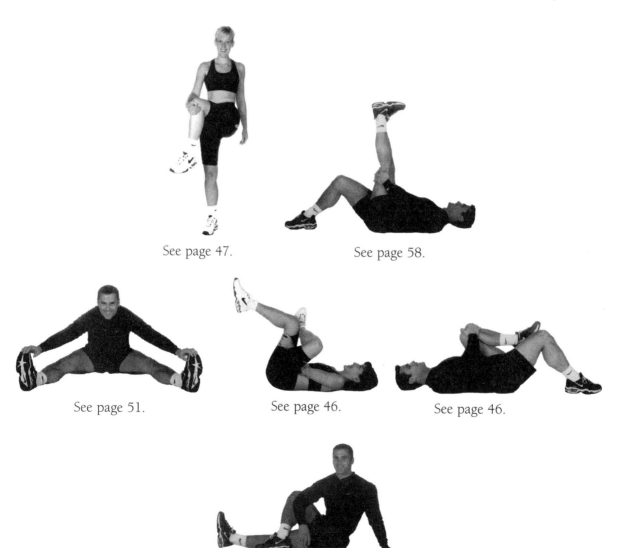

See page 47.

See page 58.

See page 51.

See page 46.

See page 46.

See page 49.

Migraine Headache

Migraines are vascular headaches in which the blood vessels of the scalp become narrow. Migraines occur from diet (simple sugars), alcohol, sunshine, stress, hormonal changes, and neck joint muscle and nerve irritation. A classic migraine usually affects one side of the head. It also involves an aura of some type with symptoms of anxiety, depression, vomiting, loss/blur-ring of vision, hearing loss, and heightened sense of smell. A common migraine can have similar symptoms, which include a throbbing pain, but typically has no aura.

Current scientific literature indicates that the nerve pathway causing migraines is the same path that produces muscle-tension headaches. Stretching, relaxation, and chiropractic care can treat migraines. In fact, some studies demonstrate that chiropractic care can reduce migraine intensity, frequency, and duration by 75–80%.

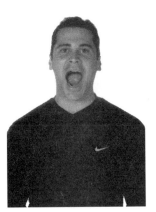
See page 29.

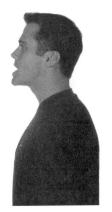
See page 29.

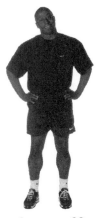
See page 32.

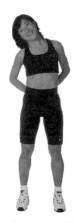
See page 32.

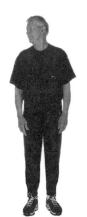
See page 31.

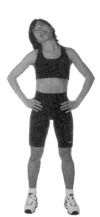
See page 33.

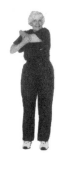
See page 35.

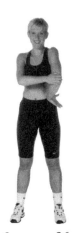
See page 36.

Muscle Tension Headache

This type of headache is caused by a contraction of the head, neck, and/or jaw muscles with or without tension (stress). Stress tends to aggravate an already preexisting condition present in these muscles and joints. It is often referred to as a "vice-grip" feeling around the head in which you experience a dull ache or pressure sensation. These headaches are often the result of poor posture.

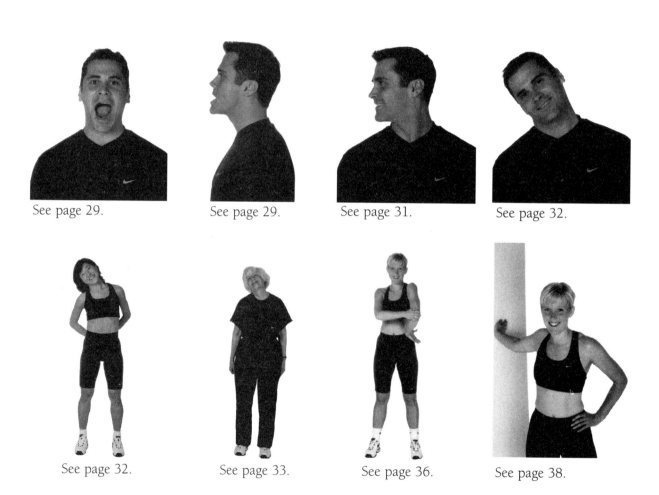

See page 29.   See page 29.   See page 31.   See page 32.

See page 32.   See page 33.   See page 36.   See page 38.

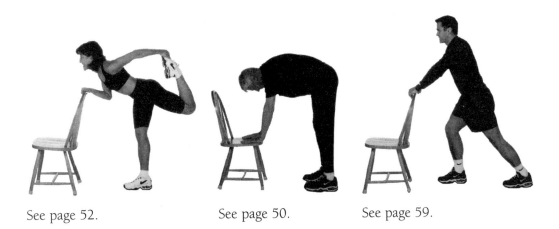

See page 52.   See page 50.   See page 59.

TMJ (Temporo-Mandibular Joint) Dysfunction

Many symptoms can arise from the malfunctioning of the joints, discs, and muscles of the jaw.

These include a reflexive muscle spasm of the jaw and other facial muscles. Clenching the jaw, grinding the teeth, dental surgery, congenital malformations, and even neck nerve irritation can cause TMJ pain. Dental, chiropractic, and massage therapy can help this common dysfunction.

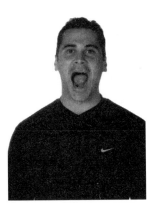

See page 29.

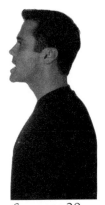

See page 29.

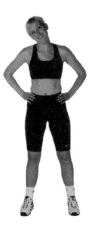

See page 32.

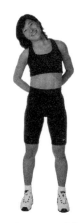

See page 32.

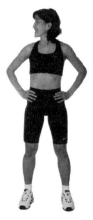

See page 31.

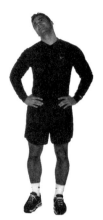

See page 33.

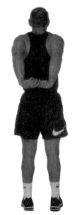

See page 40.

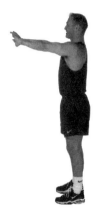

See page 34.

Carpal Tunnel Syndrome

This condition occurs from repetitive strain injury (RSI) in which the wrist tendons and forearm flexors become inflamed and thickened. The tendons become painfully trapped as they pass through the channel in the wrist formed by the hand (carpal) bones and the ligament of the hand. What makes this tunnel clinically significant is that the nerve from the neck and blood vessels (called the median nerve) passing through here can become compressed. Sometimes it is also trapped and irritated in the elbow region. Tendon inflammation from overuse or improper use squeezes these nerves and vessels to cause numbness, tingling, sweating, swelling, and severe pain.

RSI usually involves poor body posture. Neck strain and blocked nerve flow can predispose or exacerbate this condition. When the neck nerves are involved with the wrist nerve, it is referred to as "double crush" syndrome ("triple crush" when the elbow in involved) and surgery is the last option chosen to relieve it. We suggest that you consult a chiropractor for a conservative treatment first. Neck and arm stretches, proper posture, and correct ergonomics are essential to correcting and preventing this condition (see Chapter 12).

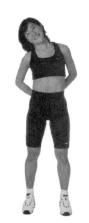

See page 32.

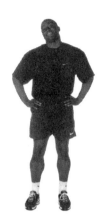

See page 33.

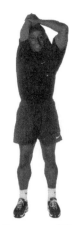

See page 35.

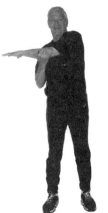

See page 36.

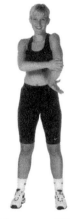

See page 36.

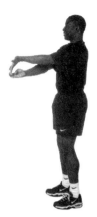

See page 44.

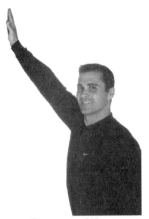

See page 37.

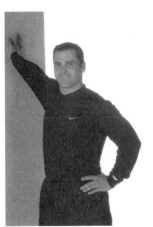

See page 36.

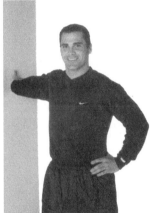

See page 38.

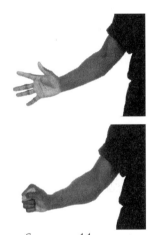

See page 44.

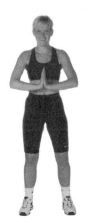

See page 42.

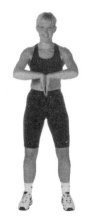

See page 42.

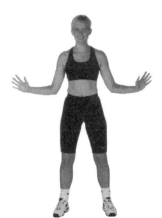

See page 43.

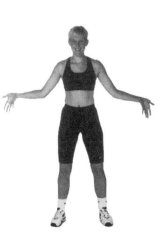

See page 43.

Stretches for Specific Occupations

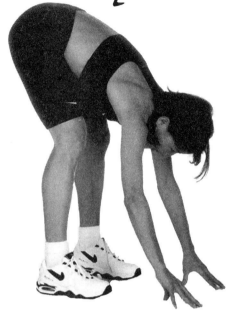

*I*t would require several volumes of text to thoroughly describe the mechanical stresses that each and every occupation places on the human body. In order to make this chapter concise and easy to follow, occupations have been organized into three sections:

1. Sitting occupations;
2. Standing occupations;
3. Bending and/or lifting occupations.

This chapter is for those who have pain or who wish to better understand the workplace stressors, how to eliminate pain, and how to prevent the effects of these stresses on the muscles and joints. Since stretches for specific pain syndromes were described in Chapter 11, let's now focus on prevention. Surprisingly, muscle stress and tension can develop from virtually any profession. As stated earlier, low back pain is one of the most common afflictions in Western society. Therefore, we must educate the two most common groups of people who suffer from this problem: heavy lifters and excessive sitters.

If you have one or more of the following warning signs, you should have a chiropractor examine your back:

1. You already have back pain and stiffness.
2. You are overweight and/or out of shape.
3. You have restricted mobility/flexibility.
4. You often slouch while standing or sitting.
5. You stand with one foot twisted out.
6. You have a short leg that causes your pelvis to tilt.

7. Your head and/or shoulders tilt.

8. Your shoes wear out on one side.

9. You lift with your back instead of your legs.

10. You twist or reach out while lifting.

Repetitive strain injuries can occur in any occupation where the same movement is done over and over again. Even occupations that involve prolonged postures or held positions can cause repetitive stress.

To use this chapter effectively, locate the category your occupation falls under and follow the appropriate preventative stretches as well as ergonomic tips. Make the necessary adjustments to you and your work area. It will make your job much easier and substantially reduce your risk of injury.

SITTING OCCUPATIONS

Improper sitting, which is most commonly caused by slouching in a chair with the knees higher than the pelvis, puts strain on the spinal column and causes disc distortion, ineffective breathing (from stress on the diaphragm), and poor digestion. Prolonged sitting can also shorten your hamstrings and lengthen your back neck muscles. The worst sitting occupations are those in which there is vibrational stress that can damage the spine (e.g., truck drivers).

Every hour of work requires a 2–6 minute stretching break. This reduces muscular fatigue, pain, and degenerative joint/disc problems, which dramatically increases work productivity. If your employer does not endorse a stretch break, suggest trying it for a month and monitoring the overall performance of your work or your group. If work efficiency increases, you can always ask for a raise!

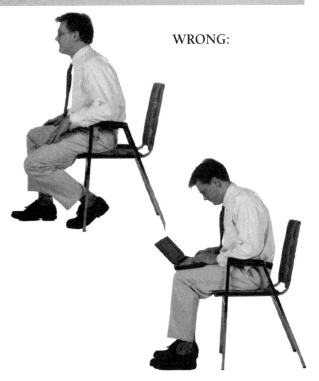

WRONG:

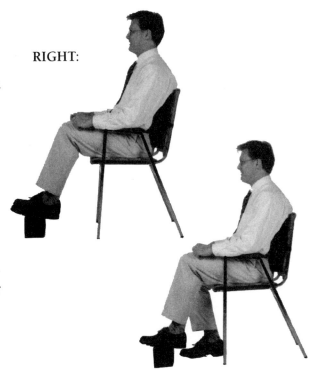

RIGHT:

Guidelines for the Computer Workstation

The Chair

1. Adjust height so that knees are horizontal to floor or slightly lower with respect to hips (see photos).
2. Maintain proper low back curve; this will help keep the upper back and neck straight. A back support for your chair can help.
3. Do not remain seated for too long. Try to get up and stretch at least once an hour.

The Desk/Keyboard

1. The upper arms should be in line with the torso.
2. The forearm should be perpendicular to the upper arm and in line with the table.
3. The hands should be in line with the forearm.

The Work Materials and Monitor Screen

1. Place materials, including documents, directly in front of you. The document that receives the most attention should be more centrally positioned.
2. Keep the top of the screen at eye level. The small muscles of the eyes will tire less quickly when looking down rather than looking up.
3. Keep the screen approximately at arm's length and at right angles to the line of sight.

Remember:

Other factors may be contributing to the problem (e.g., poor vision, poor posture, and/or highly repetitive activities). If tension builds up during the day, get up and stretch or walk around. Problems such as muscle stiffness, weakness, nerve irritation, and even headaches can arise if you do not follow the above recommendations. If you still experience discomfort after following the guidelines, consult your chiropractor.

RIGHT:

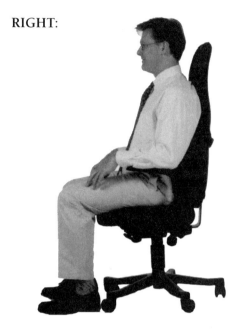

RIGHT:

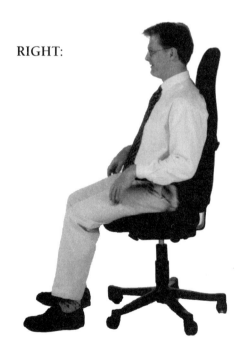

Sitting Occupation Stretches

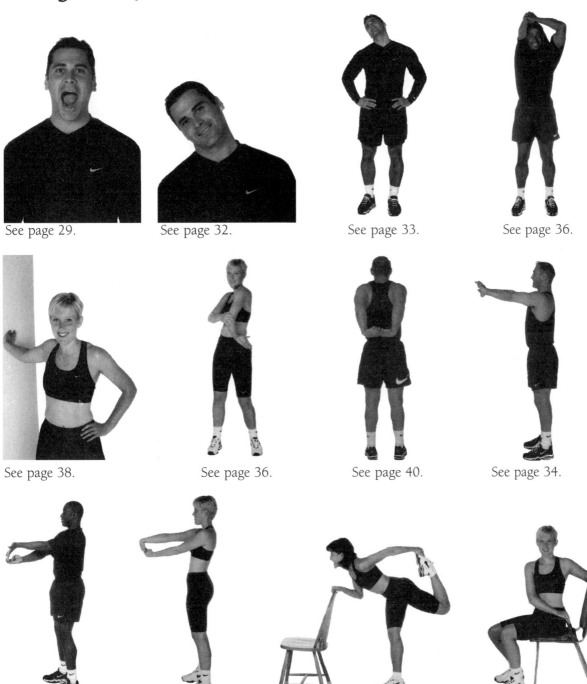

See page 29.   See page 32.   See page 33.   See page 36.

See page 38.   See page 36.   See page 40.   See page 34.

See page 44.   See page 44.   See page 52.   See page 49.

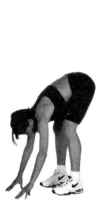
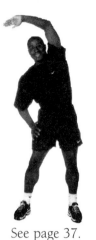
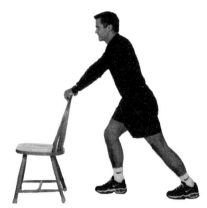
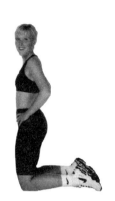

See page 50.   See page 37.   See page 59.   See page 60.

STANDING OCCUPATIONS

When you are standing, it is very easy for muscles to stiffen up, mostly from insufficient blood flow to the areas that need it. Circulation throughout the body is dependent on movement. Without continuous muscular contraction and relaxation, the "physiological pump" that pushes blood from the legs to the heart and lungs cannot be utilized to the fullest. Blood is not re-oxygenated as quickly and delivery of nutrients to working muscles is diminished. In general, stretch at least 2 minutes for every 20–30 minutes of work.

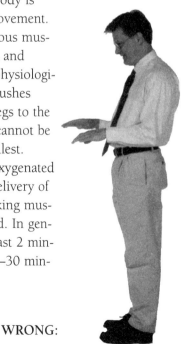

WRONG:

RIGHT:

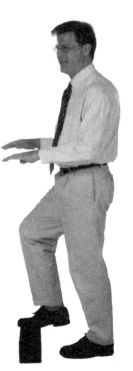

Helpful Hints When Standing:

1. Wear rubber-soled shoes for shock absorption.
2. Wear shoes with good ankle support.
3. Stand on a rubber mat.
4. Avoid concrete surfaces.
5. Raise a leg onto a stool to reduce low back strain (see photo).
6. Never completely lock your knees.

Standing Occupation Stretches

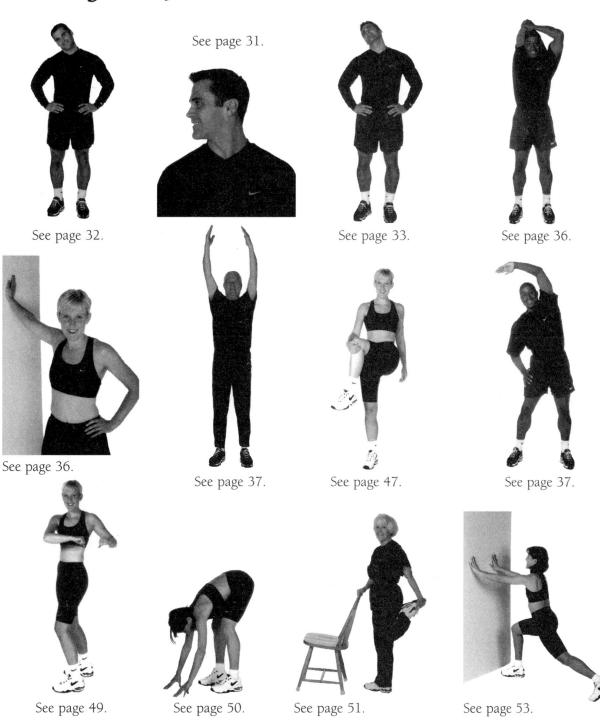

See page 31.

See page 32.

See page 33.

See page 36.

See page 36.

See page 37.

See page 47.

See page 37.

See page 49.

See page 50.

See page 51.

See page 53.

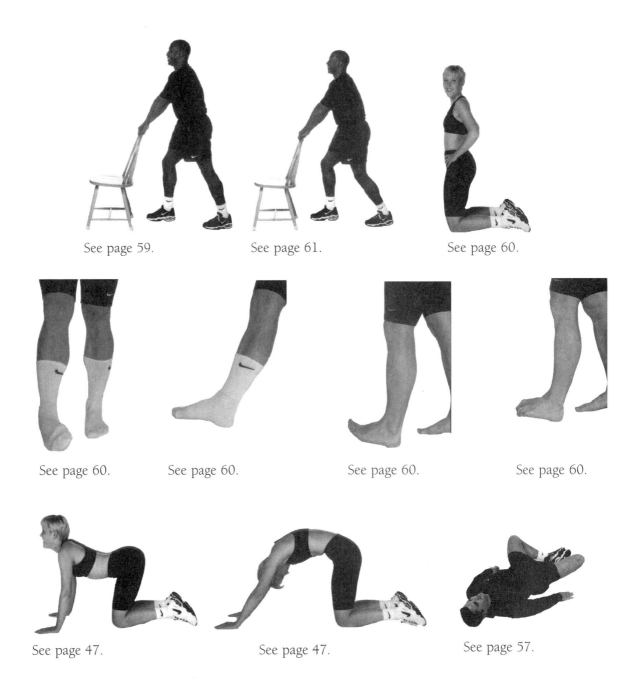

See page 59.　　　　See page 61.　　　　See page 60.

See page 60.　　See page 60.　　　　See page 60.　　　　See page 60.

See page 47.　　　　　See page 47.　　　　　See page 57.

BENDING AND LIFTING OCCUPATIONS

Bending and twisting combined with lifting is the most dangerous combination of movements because it places excessive force on the spinal discs, especially in the lower back. The result can be abnormal movement and weakening of the ligaments which hold the vertebral bones in their proper position and secure the discs that sit between the vertebrae to absorb shock. The ligaments will eventually separate from the repetitive strain. This can lead to a herniated, or bulging, disc. Anyone who has had this problem can attest to the extreme pain felt when this happens.

Helpful Hints When Lifting

1. Get close to the load.
2. Bend at the knees and hips, not at the waist.
3. Keep your shoulders above your hips and look forward (head upright). This will help maintain the spinal curves.
4. Lift with the legs and buttocks, not the back.
5. Breathe out as you lift. Do not hold your breath!
6. Lift slowly.
7. Do not twist as you lift.
8. Move your feet instead of twisting your upper body when you stand or turn.
9. Avoid overhead lifts. Use a stool or ladder.
10 Use mechanical devices or get help if the object is too heavy.
11. Remember to think before you act.

Bending and Lifting Occupation Stretches

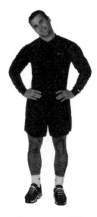 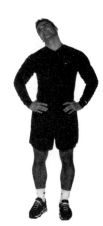 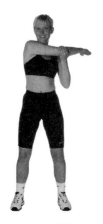 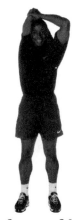

See page 32.   See page 33.   See page 35.   See page 36.

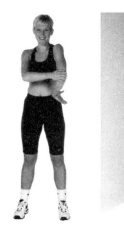 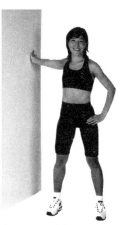 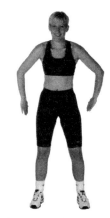 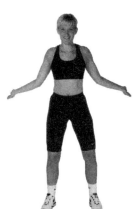 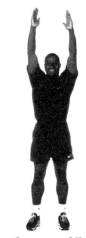

See page 36.　　See page 38.　　　　See page 35.　　　　See page 39.　　　　See page 37.

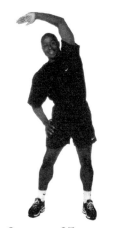 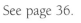 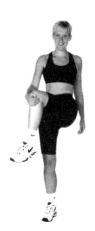 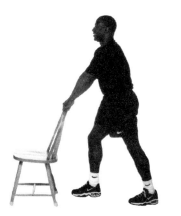 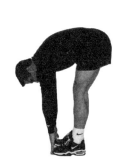

See page 37.　　　　　See page 47.　　　　See page 59.　　　　　See page 50.

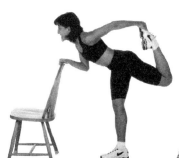 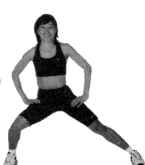 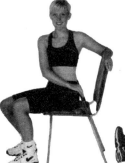 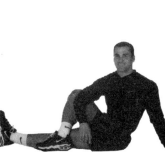

See page 52.　　　　　See page 56.　　　　See page 49.　　　　See page 49.

Household Activities: Stretches & Postures

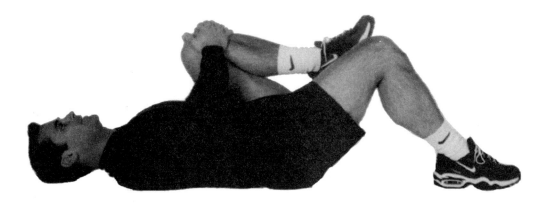

One of the most common misconceptions about household chores is that they are physically easy and require no warm-up or cool-down stretches. This is *not* the case.

FACTS

1. Household chores are one of the most common causes of strain injury seen in general practice (e.g., vacuuming causing low back pain, raking causing shoulder pain, gardening causing pelvic pain).
2. Household chores require physical work much like exercise. For the average person, household chores are much more physically demanding than those of a regular job.
3. Household chores usually require prolonged periods of work. In fact, they require more time than does your typical exercise routine (one hour). For example, raking the leaves can take 2-4 consecutive hours to complete.

The following guidelines are new and unique methods of sensibly approaching your daily household in order to help minimize the risk of injury. Included are recommended "pre-chore" warm-up stretches as well as "post-chore" cool-down stretches for each activity.

INDOOR ACTIVITIES

Child Care

Suggestions:

1. Lift even the smallest of child with your knees bent and the child close to your body.
2. Avoid twisting, particularly while holding a child when getting into a car.
3. As soon as the child can walk, give him or her as much opportunity to do so as possible.
4. If a child is crying, do not lift him or her up. Crouch down to the child's level to give a hug.

5. Use proper equipment (e.g., a changing table instead of a floor).

6. Use a lunge-type stance if the crib does not have a moveable side. Try to purchase a crib with a moveable side and the ability to change the bed's height.

7. Placing the child on one hip when carrying him or her actually increases strain on your back.

Prior to starting your day as a parent, particularly for the first 2 years of your child's life, we suggest you perform a general stretch routine as described in Chapter 8. These 2 years will involve less sleep and more lifting than the average back is used to. It is very common to see mothers and fathers suffer low back pain as well as shoulder and neck strain during the first 2 years of parenting.

Cleaning the Tub

Suggestions:

1. Never bend into the tub from the outside.
2. Climb into the tub to reduce lower back strain, especially to clean the walls, tub, and faucets.
3. Wear rubber-soled shoes to minimize the possibility of slipping.
4. Keep your center of gravity low; bend your knees or kneel down.

Do:

1. Kneel in the tub to clean all areas.
2. Stand in the tub to clean the walls.

Don't:

1. Lean over the edge of the tub to clean inside.
2. Lean in to clean tub walls.

Specific stretches for cleaning the tub:

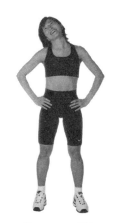

See page 33.

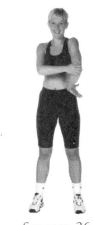

See page 36.

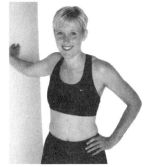

See page 38.

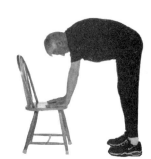

See page 50.

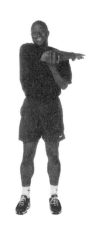

See page 35.

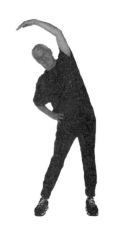

See page 37.

Dusting/Window Cleaning

Suggestions:

1. Avoid reaching.
2. Avoid bending at the waist.
3. If a ladder is required, ask for help to hold it steady.
4. Wear a belt to hold both cleaner and towel so that reaching may be avoided.
5. Kneel at waist level to avoid bending while cleaning.

Do:

1. Use two chairs instead of one to stand on.
2. Kneel instead of bending at the waist.

Don't:

1. Reach.

Specific stretches:

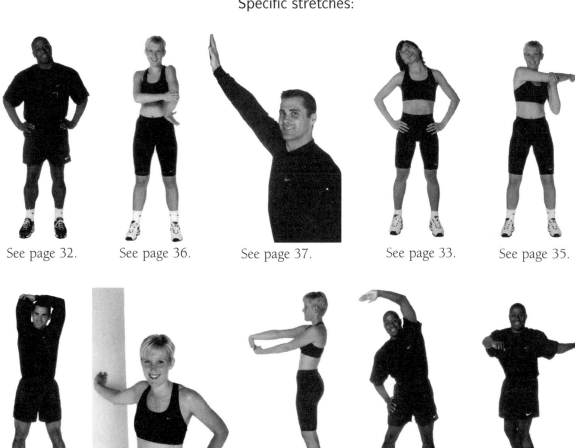

| See page 32. | See page 36. | See page 37. | See page 33. | See page 35. |

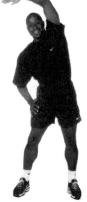
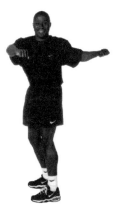

| See page 36. | See page 38. | See page 44. | See page 37. | See page 49. |

Laundry

Suggestions:

1. Do several small loads.
2. For a top-load machine, use a lunge-type stance with one arm supporting body weight.
3. For a front-load machine, bend one knee.

4. Don't put all the clothes in for a specific load at once.

Do:

1. Kneel on one knee and reach to prevent low back strain.

Don't:

1. Bend at the waist with both legs straight into the machine.

Specific stretches:

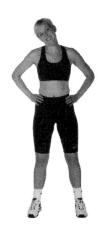

See page 32.

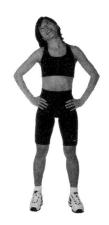

See page 33.

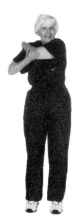

See page 35.

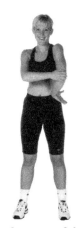

See page 36.

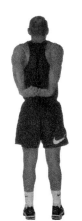

See page 40.

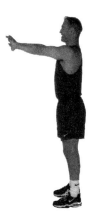

See page 34.

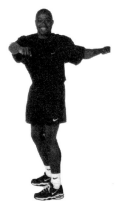

See page 49.

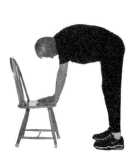

See page 50.

Making the Bed

Suggestions:

1. Work from both sides of the bed.
2. Don't bend at the waist.
3. Lift bed corners with bent knees.
4. Lean on one arm.
5. Avoid reaching across the bed; kneel on the bed if necessary.

6. When flipping your mattress, ask a friend or family member for help.
7. Don't hold your breath; this leads to lower back strain.

Do:

1. Bend at the knees to tuck the corners in.

Don't:

1. Bend at the waist and reach to tuck in corners.

Specific stretches:

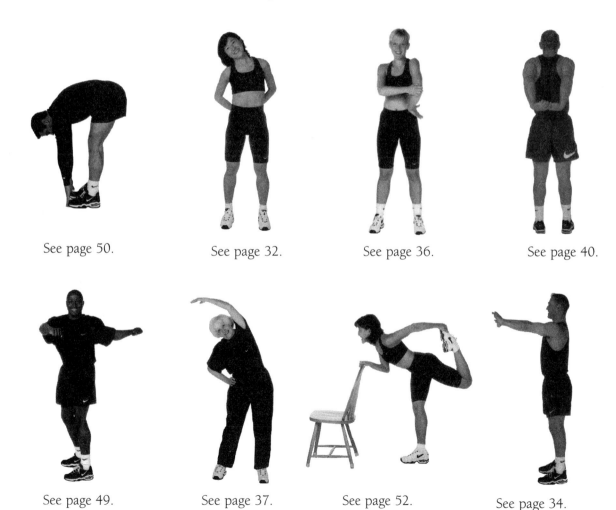

See page 50. See page 32. See page 36. See page 40.

See page 49. See page 37. See page 52. See page 34.

Painting

Suggestions:

1. Elevate the paint can to avoid bending.
2. Use a broom handle and rollers to avoid reaching.
3. Avoid excessive neck extension (i.e., leaning backwards).
4. Avoid prolonged stationary posture.
5. Take a stretch break every 20–30 minutes, since stiffness can quickly occur.

6. Do not try to rush or do too much in one day. Break up the job to avoid excessive loading to the muscles and joints.
7. Use a stool to flex the leg when standing.
8. Do 2–5 minutes of stretching for every 30 minutes of painting.

> **Painting and vacuuming without adequate stretching are the most common causes of indoor injuries.**

Specific stretches:

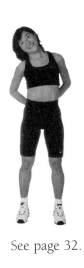

See page 32.

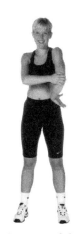

See page 36.

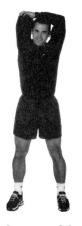

See page 36.

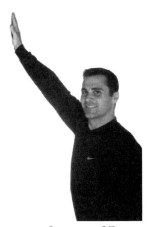

See page 37.

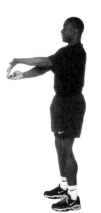

See page 44.

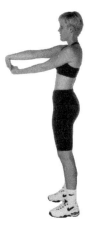

See page 44.

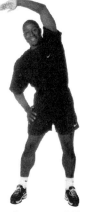

See page 37.

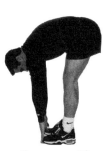

See page 50.

Vacuuming/Mopping/Waxing Floors

Suggestions:

1. Purchase the appropriate height, length, and weight of appliance. If the appliance is too short, it will cause more bending and, therefore, more chance of lower back strain.

2. Bend the knees to absorb the stress of pushing the vacuum.

3. Minimize bending at the waist.

4. Wear appropriate shoes (e.g., running shoes) for traction and shock absorption.

5. Minimize twisting at the waist to reduce stress to lower back discs.

6. Move your feet; keep them shoulder-width apart.

7. Kneel on one knee to vacuum under furniture. Keep your back straight; lean on one arm if necessary.

8. If you have a lower back problem, avoid vacuuming; it will exacerbate the symptoms.

9. Rock your pelvis back and forth.

10. Walk with the vacuum; pulling it toward you can strain the lower back.

11. Avoid scrubbing floors on your hands and knees. Use a mop handle.

Do:

1. Walk through the activity, do not rush.

2. Flex the front knee as you push.

Don't:

1. Bend at the waist.

> **Vacuuming and painting without adequate stretching are the most common causes of indoor injuries.**

Specific stretches:

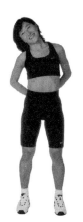 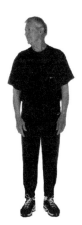 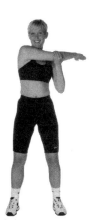 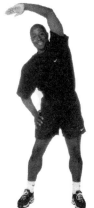 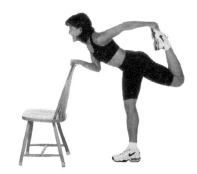

See page 32.   See page 31.   See page 35.   See page 37.   See page 52.

OUTDOOR ACTIVITIES

Lawn Cutting

Suggestions:

1. Keep your head up.
2. Avoid bending at the waist.

3. Avoid pushing to the side of the mower or with one hand.
4. Stand directly behind the mower.
5. Keep your hips and shoulders in line with your spine.
6. Avoid pulling the mower uphill. It is much easier to push uphill.
7. Avoid twisting or lifting the mower.

Specific stretches:

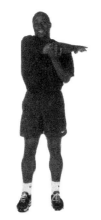 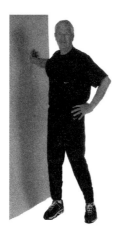 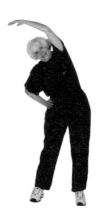 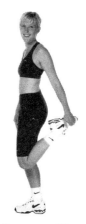

See page 35. See page 38. See page 37. See page 51.

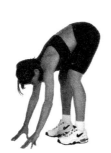 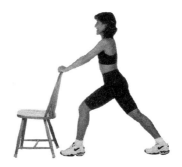

See page 50. See page 59.

Gardening

Suggestions:

1. Avoid bending at the waist.
2. Bend on one knee.
3. If you have a knee problem, you can sit on a stool or lie down.

4. Avoid pulling up roots from a standing position; don't hold your breath.
5. Avoid twisting.
6. Avoid prolonged postures involving the lower back and neck, as they are common sites for strain.
7. Use a long-handled hoe wherever possible.

Specific stretches:

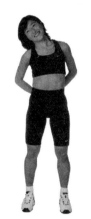
See page 32.

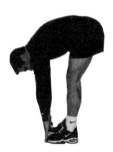
See page 37.

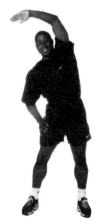
See page 50.

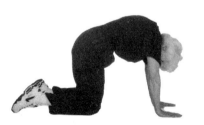
See page 47.

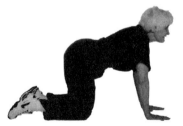
See page 47.

Lifting Garbage

Suggestions:

1. Bend your knees.
2. Keep the bag light.
3. Don't twist.
4. Keep the bag close to your body when lifting it into a pail.

Do:

1. Bend knees.

Don't:

1. Twist at the waist; this can lead to disc injury.

Specific stretches:

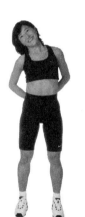

See page 32.

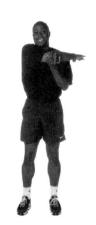

See page 35.

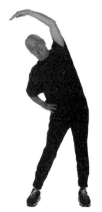

See page 37.

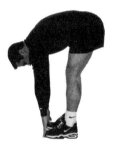

See page 50.

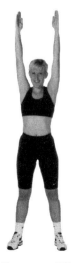

See page 37.

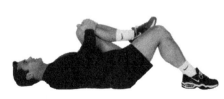

See page 46.

Raking

Suggestions:

1. Hold the rake with one hand at shoulder height, one hand at waist height.
2. Bend at the knees, not at the waist.
3. Walk with the pile of leaves. Do not pull at the waist.
4. Wear gloves.

5. Take a break every 30–45 minutes to prevent injuries.

Do:

1. Drag the leaves while walking.

Don't:

1. Bend or twist, especially with a large pile of leaves.

Specific stretches:

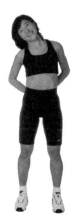

See page 32.

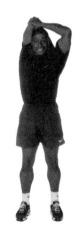

See page 36.

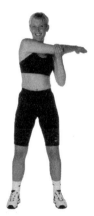

See page 35.

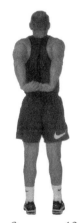

See page 40.

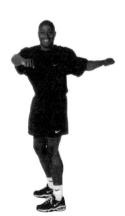

See page 49.

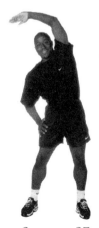

See page 37.

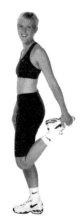

See page 51.

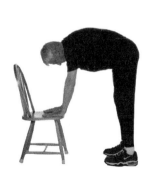

See page 50.

Shoveling Snow

This is the most common cause of outdoor injuries.

Suggestions:

1. Do not shovel snow if you have lower back pain!

2. Bend your knees to lift. Push the snow forward. Lift smaller loads of wet snow.

3. Keep the snow close to your body.

4. Do not bend at the waist. Always bend at the knees.

5. Wear boots with treads to decrease the possibility of slippage.

6. Avoid weight belts. If the snow is too heavy, avoid this task.

7. Hold the handle with one hand and place the other hand as close to the shovel scoop as possible before lifting.

8. An ergonomic shovel with a bent handle reduces the amount of bending and prevents back injury. Better yet, hire a young person to clear snow.

Do:

1. Bend your knees to lift.

Don't:

1. Twist.

Specific stretches:

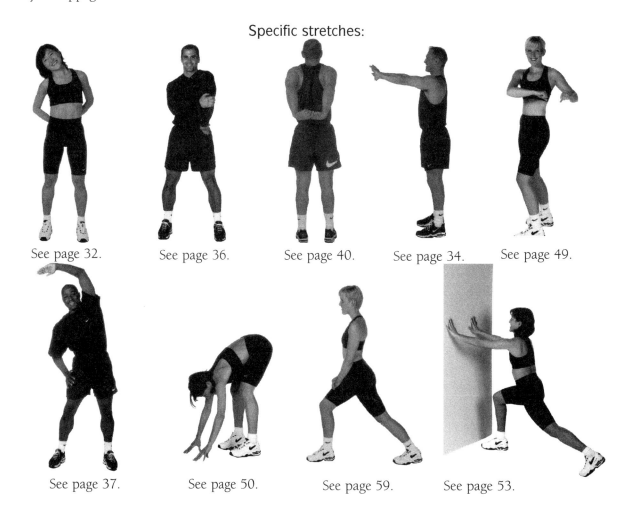

See page 32. See page 36. See page 40. See page 34. See page 49.

See page 37. See page 50. See page 59. See page 53.

Unloading From Vehicle

Suggestions:

1. Avoid leaning with groceries into the back seat unless this can be done in a walk-in level truck.
2. Use the trunk to avoid bending into the car.
3. Place one knee on the trunk bumper to lift.
4. Carry only what you can lift—no more. This will reduce neck and shoulder strain.

Do:
1. Use the knee for support.

Don't:
1. Bend at the waist and lean into the trunk.

Specific stretches:

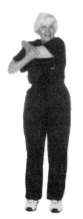

See page 35.

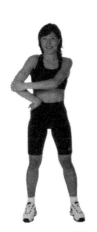

See page 36.

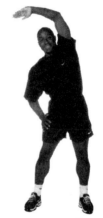

See page 37.

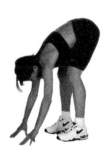

See page 50.

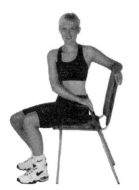

See page 49.

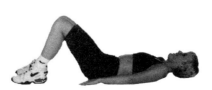

See page 48.

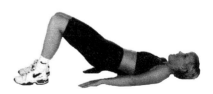

See page 48.

171

Stretching for Pregnancy & Delivery

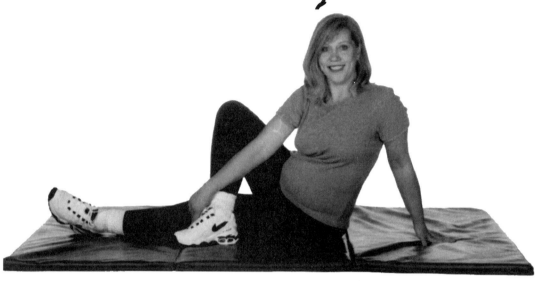

A woman undergoes many physical, mental, and lifestyle changes during and after pregnancy. It is important that she has proper exercise and nutrition, and engages in stretching before, during, and after giving birth.

Stretching and exercising help pregnant women in many ways. They improve circulation, help digestion, aid elimination, reduce stress, enhance restful sleep, increase energy, improve mood, limit weight gain, and reduce fatigue/shortness of breath. They also better prepare the pelvic muscles for a greater tolerance to the discomfort during childbirth. Greater flexibility improves posture, muscle strength and tone, which reduces joint and ligament strain. Exercise can also help strengthen muscles as well as regulate body metabolism and temperature.

Since there are so many benefits to stretching and exercise, one may question why more preg-

nant women do not to take part in fitness regimes. This chapter is presented in three sections for the first and second halves of pregnancy as well as postpartem (after) delivery. We do not mention of pre-pregnancy, because we assume you are already enjoying optimal health with the help from the first eight-chapters of this book. If not, it is something you may want to engage in for some time before becoming pregnant.

The first part of this chapter discusses the first and second trimester (the first 6 months of pregnancy). The second part discusses the third trimester (last 3–4 months). For the first 6 months of pregnancy, your activity level can remain fairly normal. The majority of weight gain does not typically occur until the final trimester. It is also important to remember that the body undergoes additional changes after delivery. The effects of sleep deprivation, breast feeding, and caring for the child take their toll.

Women who do not regularly exercise before pregnancy should consult their obstetrician or chiropractor before beginning an exercise routine. Start at a very low intensity level.

If you have exercised prior to becoming pregnant, you should still exercise regularly when pregnant. Many bodily changes are occurring:

1. Hormones, such as relaxin, are released to help your joints and ligaments stretch with delivery. If you engage in pounding or high impact exercises, like running or aerobics, you seriously risk straining the pelvic joints and weakening the pelvic floor tissues, which may increase your chances of low back pain.

2. During the second trimester, the uterus enlarges and presses on the inferior vena cava (a large vein that returns blood from the lower body to the heart). If you perform exercises or stretches on your back, you can restrict the return of blood to the heart. This may cause increased blood pressure and promote swelling in the legs. Standing, sitting, or side lying movements are suggested. Blood volume increases by 30–55% during pregnancy, which can strain the cardiovascular system.

3. As your body weight increases, particularly in the abdominal area, your center of gravity changes. The baby pulls the body forward, which causes a swayback. The joints of the low back jam together to cause inflammation and pain. The knees hyperextend or lock to counteract the forward pull of the body. This leads to a tightness in the hamstrings and calves to produce leg cramps and low-back nerve irritation. The shoulders also lean backward to compensate for the baby's forward pull. This can cause contraction of the shoulder blade muscles, which yields pain in the neck and shoulder joints. The end result is a head-forward posture and a neck tilt to balance the body.

4. The stomach muscles separate as the baby grows. Do not perform any stomach exercises, such as sit-ups and crunches. Isometric exercises are good to do at this phase.

MOST COMMON SYMPTOMS FELT DURING PREGNANCY

Low Back Pain

About 56% of pregnant women experience low back pain in one to three areas: the buttocks, the base of the spine, and the waistline and/or 5 inches above it. It is usually the result of strain to the spinal joints. If the pain is sharp, there is likely to be nerve compression, which can spread to the legs and feet. This can be serious and may require you to consult your chiropractor as soon as possible. If the pain is dull, we suggest ice packs and intermittent stretching for 2 days. If the pain still persists, call your doctor or chiropractor. Spinal adjustments throughout pregnancy are safe and can help prevent pain.

Sciatica (referred pain in the legs)

1. Sciatica is compression of the low back nerves that causes electrical, or shooting, pain from the low back or buttocks to the legs and feet. If this pain begins early in pregnancy, it is likely to persist or get worse. If you have a history of this pain before pregnancy, consult your chiropractor before it worsens.

2. Referred pain is caused by nerve irritation in the lumbar and pelvis. The symptoms are aches, numbness, and/or tingling into the groin, legs, and feet. This problem is typically easier to correct than sciatica through spinal adjustment and massage therapy.

Cramping or Spasms in the Calves/Arches of the Feet

Three things can cause this symptom: 1. nerve irritation in the pelvis or low back; 2. reduced blood flow to the legs from the fetus pressing on the arteries and veins in the pelvis; 3. deficiency in calcium, magnesium, or potassium.

Pain Between the Shoulder Blades

A shortening in the upper back muscles causes a reduced blood flow (or fuel supply) to the tissues. Without oxygen, the muscle cannot perform its job effectively and becomes fatigued so that irritability, soreness, and stiffness sets in. Over time, the ribs that are attached to the spine in this area may become "misaligned" at their joints. This causes nerve irritation so that the woman feels pain through the chest, or around the chest and in the armpit.

Neck Tension

This occurs in the front and back of the neck. The front neck muscles strain in the same way as do the shoulder blade muscles previously mentioned. They shorten as the body naturally shifts the head forward to offset the backward shoulder movement. The back neck muscles suffer a continual "lengthening" strain, which weakens it and reduces blood supply to the tissues so that soreness soon follows.

Heartburn or Nausea

This is very common during pregnancy. Some authorities feel that an elevated progesterone level in early pregnancy is responsible for an accelerated emptying of the stomach so that nausea occurs later in pregnancy. Heartburn is also very common because the baby pushes up on the stomach. Consequently, the stomach becomes smaller. Food and stomach acid is forced up into the esophagus (the tube that brings food from the mouth into the stomach), and heartburn occurs. Heartburn and nausea may also be triggered by nerve irritation from between the shoulder blades. Since the nerves between the shoulder blades connect the stomach to the brain, any irritation in the middle back can cause stomach discomfort.

STRETCHES FOR EACH PHASE OF PREGNANCY

It is clear from analyzing these six most common symptoms during pregnancy that muscles, tendons, nerves, and joints are the common denominators. The best kinds of stretching for these aches and pains are slow, static stretches.

To follow are stretches that you can do for each phase of pregnancy. They need to be performed one to three times a day. They will help relieve the discomfort from the stress on the muscles, bones, and joints as well as the intensity, frequency, and duration of pregnancy symptoms.

As pregnancy progresses, the majority of the standing stretches should ideally be performed in a swimming pool. The buoyancy of the water substantially reduces the effects of gravity on the joints and muscles, which helps to lessen pain and stiffness.

Phase 1: 0–6 Months

Standing Stretches

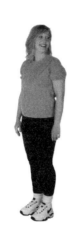

See page 32.

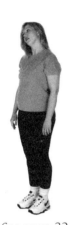

See page 31.

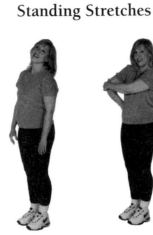

See page 33.

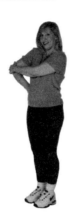

See page 36.

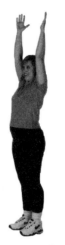

See page 37.

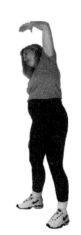

See page 37.

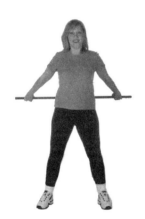

See page 40.

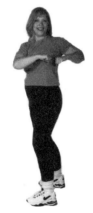

See page 49.

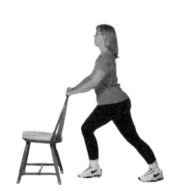

See page 59.

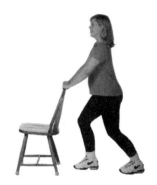

See page 61.

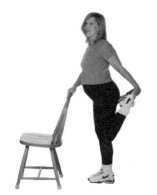

See page 51.

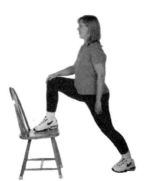

See page 53.

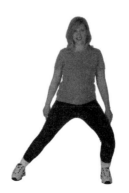

See page 56.

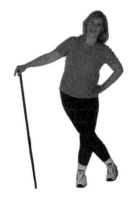

See page 48.

Sitting Stretches

Sitting on a chair is the most comfortable and easiest position to rise from while carrying the extra weight during pregnancy.

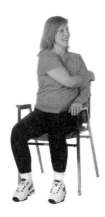

See page 49.

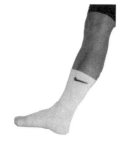

See page 60.

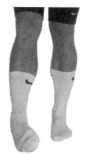

See page 60.

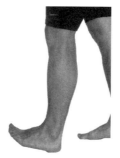

See page 60.

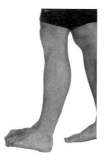

See page 60.

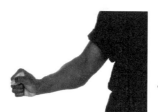

See page 44.

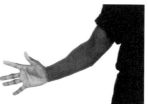

See page 44.

Floor Stretches

The neck stretches can be done standing, sitting, or resting on the floor.

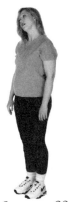

See page 32.

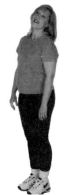

See page 31.

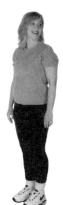

See page 33.

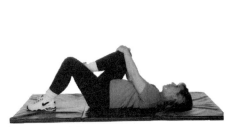

See page 46.

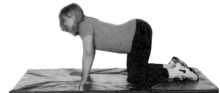

See page 47.

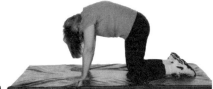

See page 47.

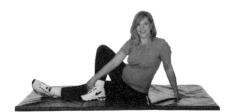

See page 49.

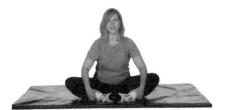

See page 57.

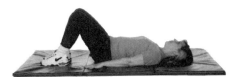

See page 48.

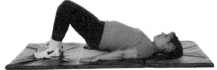

See page 48.

Phase 2: 6–10 Months

Standing Stretches

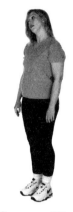

See page 32.

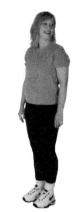

See page 31.

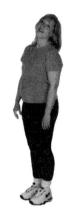

See page 33.

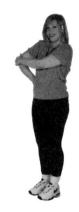

See page 36.

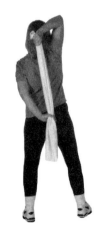

See page 34.

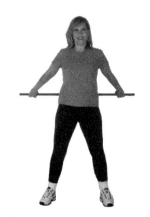

See page 40.

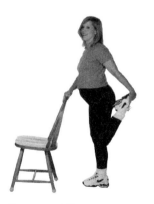

See page 51.

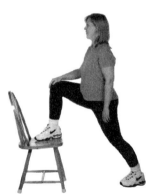

See page 53.

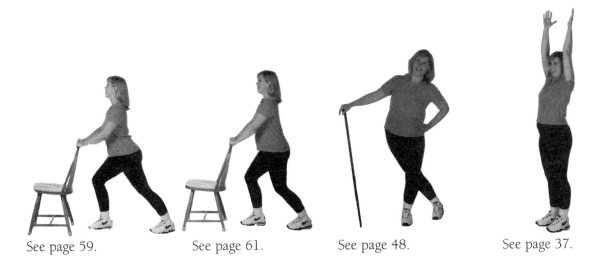

See page 59.   See page 61.   See page 48.   See page 37.

Sitting Stretches

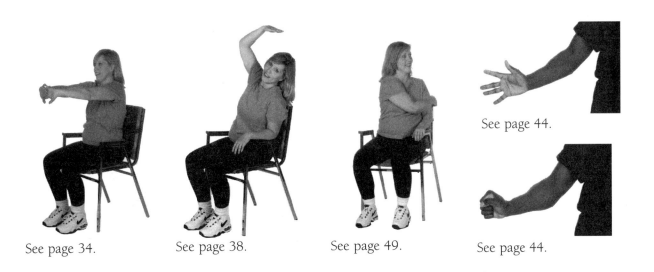

See page 34.   See page 38.   See page 49.   See page 44.

See page 44.

Floor Stretches

During the second phase of pregnancy, you should avoid lying on your back, because it often causes heartburn and reduces blood flow to and from the heart. It is also a difficult position to rise from with out assistance. We suggest that you avoid *excessive* extension of the spine, as pregnancy already places a great deal of extension stress on the joints of the lower back.

See page 47. 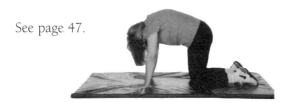 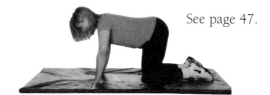 See page 47.

Phase 3: Post-Pregnancy

Standing Stretches

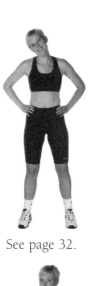 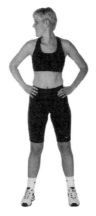 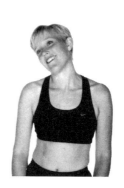 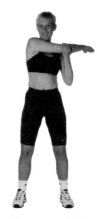

See page 32.   See page 31.   See page 33.   See page 35.

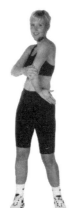 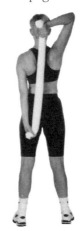 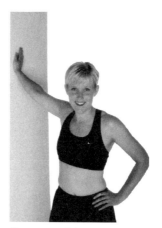 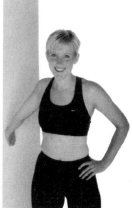

See page 36.   See page 34.   See page 36.   See page 39.

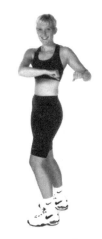

See page 49.

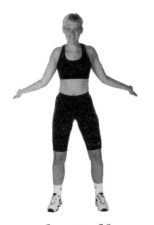

See page 39.

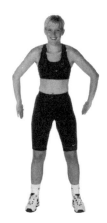

See page 35.

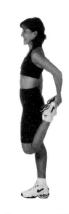

See page 51.

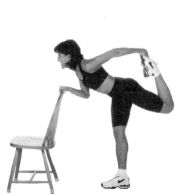

See page 52.

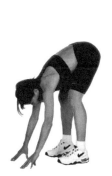

See page 58.

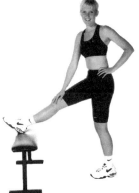

See page 50.

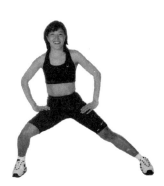

See page 56.

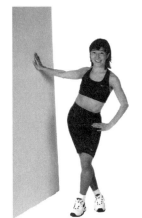

See page 48.

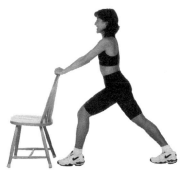

See page 59.

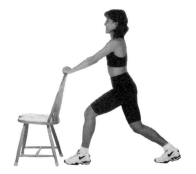

See page 61.

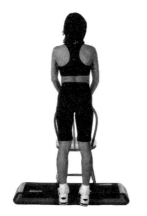

See page 61.

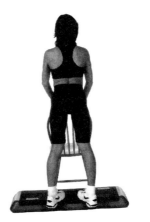

See page 61.

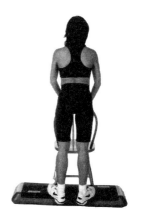

See page 61.

Sitting Stretches

Floor Stretches

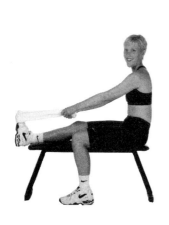

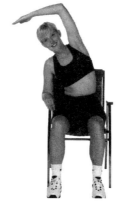

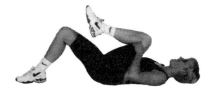

See page 46.

See page 54.

See page 38.

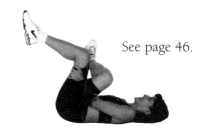

See page 46.

See page 51.

See page 51.

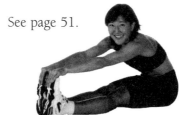

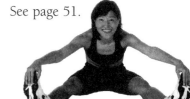

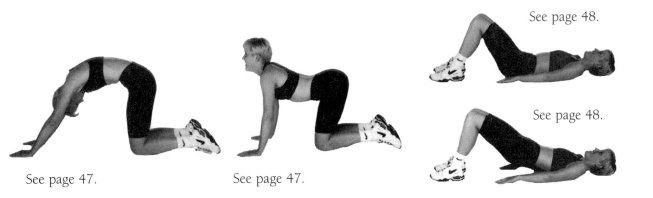

See page 48.

See page 48.

See page 47.

See page 47.

Exercise Recommendations for Pregnancy

1. Exercise moderately and regularly three to five times a week.

2. Reduce workout intensity by 25%.

3. Stick to non-weight bearing exercises, such as stationary bike, aquatics (water aerobics), and swimming. Spend additional time warming up, stretching, and cooling down.

4. Avoid high-impact activities, especially ones in which you could fall.

5. If weight training, use lighter weights and do more repetitions.

6. Avoid bouncing movements, jumping, jarring, quick directional changes, and deep forward or backward bends.

7. Do not exercise on your back.

8. Avoid excessive heat and humidity. Stay out of hot tubs, saunas, and so on. Drink plenty of water before, during, and after exercising.

9. Eat plenty of complex carbohydrates (pasta, rice, whole grain products). This is good for anyone who exercises regularly.

10. Always listen to your body. Stop exercising if you feel faint, dizzy, or if any unusual symptoms occur. Consult your physician immediately.

Exercises for the Abdomen & Low Back

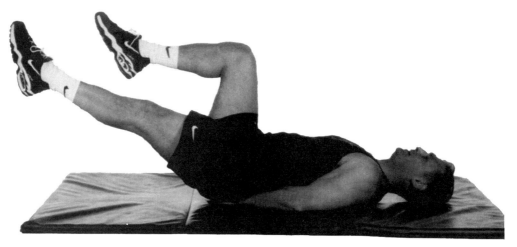

*E*xercise can be confusing. Your doctor may say one thing, your aerobics trainer may say another, and this book says something else. Regardless of what area of the body you are exercising, you should always use your own common sense first. In general, you are ready to exercise after 1 or 2 months of perfecting your stretching technique. Think about the exercise you are doing and how it relates to your inherent blueprint (see Chapter 5). Exercise should not cause extreme discomfort or pain if you have properly stretched before and after an exercise routine. It should make you feel good! Do not simply copy what others are doing around you particularly if it doesn't seem right. And do not start exercising when you are experiencing any stiffness, spasms, or pain of any kind.

Since stretching and exercising are so closely related, we feel that we should devote a chapter to the correct way to exercise. Exercising incorrectly can cause an accelerated breakdown of any weakened tissue (muscle, ligament, or cartilage). Thus, it would be distressing to do the correct stretches followed by the wrong exercises. The exercises in this chapter focus on the abdomen and low back. The abdomen is one of the areas that most people work on while the low back is one of the areas in which most people have discomfort. These areas are essential to us because they keep us upright. Recent studies on exercise physiology showed that wrong movements can actually have bad effects on other areas of your body. For example, incorrect stomach exercises can actually cause low back pain in addition to stomach strain. Since so many people have been doing incorrect abdomen and back exercises for years, we feel it is important for you to know the ones that you should do. By taking the time to relearn the basics, you can reach new heights with your overall health.

Safe and Effective Abdominal Exercises

Full Sit-up

Bend knees.

Keep feet flat on the floor.

Elevate hands beside the face. Do not pull the head up.

Start with the head on floor. Exhale on the rise.

Inhale at the top.

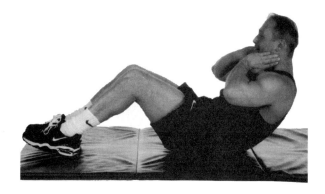

Exhale on the descent. While descending slowly, round out the spine and lower yourself one vertebrae at a time. Concentrate on the stomach muscles.

Always touch the head to the floor to reduce neck muscle strain.

Rest for 1–2 seconds before you begin again.

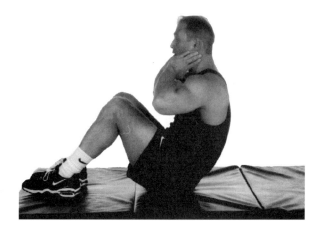

Begin with as many sit-ups as you are comfortable with and increase the number of repetitions each time. Work up to twenty-five to fifty repetitions for at least three times per week. Increase from one to three sets. This exercise is excellent for the upper and lower abdomen.

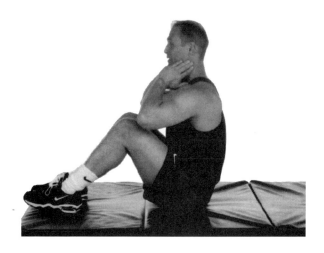

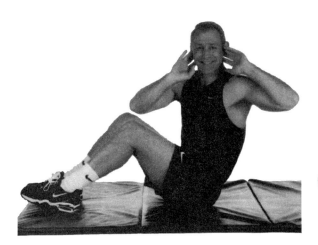

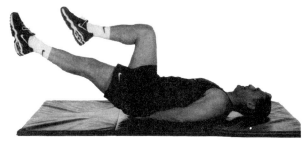

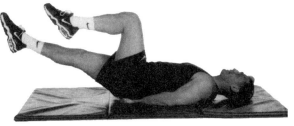

Full Sit-up with a Twist

This is the same as a full sit-up except, while rising, twist the torso slowly to the right; touch the left elbow to the right knee only if there is no pain or strain.

Inhale as you return to center.

Exhale on the descent to the floor.

Repeat with a twist to the left, following the same guidelines.

Repeat twenty to fifty times for at least three times a week. Increase from one to three sets. This exercise works the upper and lower abdominal muscles as well as side muscles.

Lying Cycle Kick

Lie flat on your back.

Clench your fists and place them under each buttock to ensure that your lower back stays flat on the ground.

Bend your knees up.

Lift your feet off the ground.

Extend the right leg with your toe pointed out straight (heel approximately 6 inches above the ground).

As you are returning the right leg to the bent position, slowly extend the left leg with the toe pointed.

This is one repetition.

Repeat twenty-five to two hundred times; slowly build up every second day, or three times a week. Increase from one to three sets. This exercise strengthens and tones the lower abdomen and upper thigh muscles. If you experience a "clicking" sound in your hip, stretch your Psoas or hip flexor muscles (see p. 50). The clicking is generally not a sign of arthritis.

Hanging Knee-to-Chest Raise

Use both hands to hold onto the bar.

Make sure that your feet do not touch the ground to ensure a full abdominal-muscle stretch.

Exhale as you raise both knees to your chest slowly.

Inhale on the descent.

Repeat ten to fifteen times every second day. Increase from one to three sets. If possible, use a health club's specialized equipment that supports your elbows while allowing you to pull your knees to chest; it will reduce shoulder strain. This exercise is excellent for the entire abdomen, in particular the lower abdomen.

Hanging Side-Leg Raise with a Twist

Same as hanging knee-to-chest raise.

Raise your legs together with bent knees. Aim the right knee toward the left side of your chest/shoulder.

Exhale on the rise.

Hold 1–2 seconds.

Inhale while descending.

Repeat with the left knee aiming toward the right side of your chest/shoulder.

Repeat ten to fifteen times every second day. Increase from one to three sets. This pattern of breathing reduces strain on the lower back. This is also good for the lower abdomen.

Abdominal-Roller Device

The abdominal-roller sit-up device can reduce neck strain. It takes a little practice to learn not to use your neck muscles and, instead, to push your head up with your arms. Doing sit-ups with this kind of device helps your upper and lower abdomen. Remember to stretch your neck and abs into extension before and after to reduce the "C" or rounding-forward posture (see p. 188, isometric extension exercise).

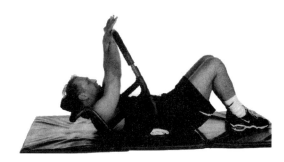

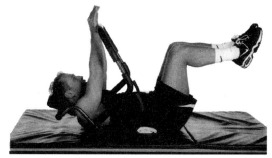

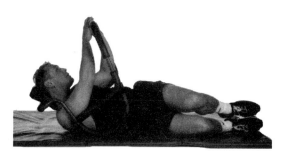

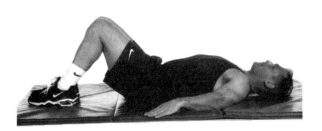

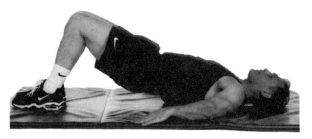

Pelvic Raises

Lie on your back with palms flat on the floor.

Bend your knees.

Keep your head on the floor.

Raise your buttocks 1–2 inches off the floor.

Hold for 5 seconds while exhaling.

Descend while inhaling.

Repeat five to ten times daily. As the stomach strengthens, continue with the lying cycle kick. Increase from one to three sets. This exercise is terrific for those who have a lower back problem and wish to slowly rebuild the stomach muscles.

Safe and Effective Low Back Exercises

Isometric Extension Exercises

Lie on your stomach.

Prop yourself up on your elbows.

Arch your back without force or hyperextension.

Hold for 5 seconds while exhaling.

Relax forward 2 inches while inhaling.

Increase from one to three sets.

Avoid this exercise if:

1. You have lower back pain (around the joints). This posture may aggravate your condition.
2. You suffer from sciatica symptoms (pinched lower back nerves) in which leg pain shoots from your lower back down the legs.
3. You have numbness or tingling sensations in your legs or feet.

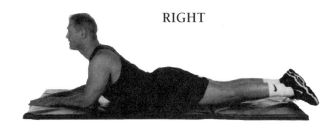

RIGHT

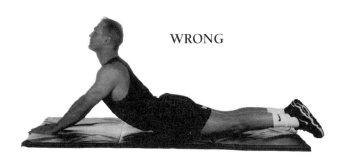

WRONG

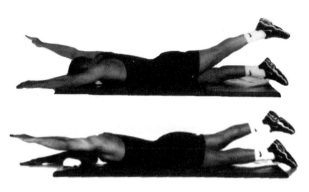

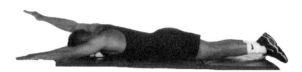

Prone Alternating Arm Raises

This exercise is the same as the prone alternating arm and leg raise except that you only raise the left arm, hold for 5–10 seconds, and then lower it.

Raise the right arm, hold for 5–10 seconds, and then lower it.

This is one repetition.

Work from five to ten repetitions. Increase from one to three sets. This exercise is good for strengthening upper back muscles. It is excellent for seniors and people with low back problems.

Prone Alternating Leg Raises

Prone Alternating Arm and Leg Raises

Lie on your stomach on the floor-not on the bed, as it is too soft. A soft surface can lead to arching of the back, which places stress on the joints.

Place a small pillow under your forehead to elevate your nose from the floor so that you can breathe. Do not turn your head to the side to perform this exercise, because you may strain your neck.

Extend your arms straight out beyond your head.

Simultaneously raise your right arm and left leg 4–6 inches off the floor. Hold for 5–10 seconds while breathing regularly. Lower your arm and leg.

Repeat on the left arm and right leg.

This is one repetition.

Start slowly and work up to five to ten repetitions, three times a week. Increase from one to three sets. This exercise strengthens the upper/lower back, buttock muscles, and back shoulder muscles. It is excellent for rehabilitation of the lower back and prevention of back pain.

NOTE: You can do any of the alternating moves standing while facing a wall. They will improve postural muscles and posture. They are excellent exercises to do on work breaks, especially if your work involves a great deal of sitting or lifting.

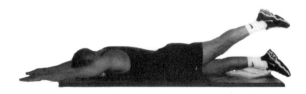

This exercise is the same as the prone alternating arm and leg raise except that you only raise the left leg, hold for 5–10 seconds, and then lower it.

Raise the right leg, hold for 5–10 seconds, and then lower it.

This is one repetition.

Work from five to ten repetitions. Increase from one to three sets. This exercise strengthens the lower back muscles.

Index

NOTE: *Boldface page numbers denote main explanation of stretch*

Abdomen
exercises, 184–188
muscles, 55
pain, 56
stretches, 55
Abdominal-Roller Device, 187
Achilles tendonitis, 128
Adductor magnus, 56
Adolescents, 17
Adults, 18
Ankle Reach, **51**, 58
Ankle sprains, 129
Arm
muscles, 41, 42
numbness, 45
Raises, Prone Alternating, 189
Arm Over Head Stretch, 36, 41
Arm Raises, Prone Alternating, 189
Asthma, 130–131

Back
harmful stretches, 69–70
low (*See* Low back)
muscles, 45, 50
stretches, 46, 50–54
warning signs for, 150–151
Back Arch, **47**, 55
Back Roll, 69
Badminton, 79–80
Ballistic (bouncing) stretching, 9, 27
Bar Chest Stretch, 40, 41
Baseball, 81–82
Basketball, 82–83
Bathtub cleaning, 160
Bed making, 163
Bending/lifting occupations, 157–158
Bent-Knee Calf Stretch, **61**
Bent Over Figure 4, 71
Biceps, 38, 41
Biceps femoris, 50, 58
Biking, 92–94
Bodybuilding, 125–126
Bottom of Wrist Stretch, **43**
Bouncing (ballistic stretching), 9, 27
Bow Posture, 73
Boxing, 84–85
Brachioradialis, 41
Break, stretches for, 12, 19, 22
Breathing, 27
Bridge Posture, 72
Bursitis, 138–139

Calcium, dietary, 20–21

Calf
muscles, 58, 61, 62
spasms/cramping, 174
strain, 128
stretches, 59–62, 61
Calf Stretch on a Step, **61**
Canoeing, 86
Cardio kickboxing, 84–85
Carpal tunnel syndrome, 148–149
Cat Stretch, **47**
Chair Lunge, **53**, 55, 56
Chair Touch, **50**, 58
Chest, 40–41
Childbirth, 13–14
Child care, 159–160
Children, 14–16
Chiropractor, 23–24, 150
Cleaning chores, 160–161
Climbing, 87–89
Closed Hand Stretch, **44**
Cold therapy, 24–25
Colic, 14
Computer workstation, guidelines for, 152
Congenital torticollis, 14
Cool-downs, 9–10
Cricket, 81–82
Cross-bridges, 20
Cross-country skiing, 91–92
Cross-legged Back Stretch, 69
Crunches, 68
Crunches with Twist, 68
Curling, 89–90
Cycling, 92–94

Dangerous movements, 67–74
Deltoid, 34, 35, 38
Deltoid Stretch, 35
Depression, postpartum, 11
Diet, 20–22
Double-Knee Crush, 71, 74
Dusting, 161
Dynamic Body Extension, 74
Dynamic work, 10

Elbow
golfer's, 134–135
tennis, 135–136
Elderly, 18–19, 65
Emotional stress, 11
Endorphin theory, 25
Enkephalins, 25
Erb's palsy, 14
Erector spinae, 45
Exercise
abdominal, 184–188
low back, 188–189
pain and, 25
during pregnancy, 172–173
vs. stretching, 8
Extensor digitorum, 42, 59
Extensor hallucis, 59
External abdominal oblique, 55
External Rotation Stretch, 40, 41

Extreme Neck Extension, 68
Extreme T-Stretch, **52**, 55, 56
Extrinsic range of motion, 75–76

Field hockey, 102–104
Figure Four Stretch, **46–47**
Flexibility
improving, 17, 18, 19
vs. stretching, 8
Flexor digitorum, 42
Flexor profundus, 42
Floors, mopping/waxing floors, 165
Floor Touch, **50–51**, 58
Foods, 21, 22
Football, 97–98
Foot Behind Head Posture, 72
Foot in Groin Hamstring Stretch, 68
Foot spasms/cramping, 174
Force, for stretching, 26
Forearm, 42
Forward Split, 73
Frog Position, 72
Front Press Out, **34**, 35, 38, 45
Frozen shoulder, 133
Full Sit-up, 185
Full Sit-up with Twist, 186

Garbage, lifting, 168
Gardening, 167
Gastrocnemius, 58, 61
"Gate" theory of pain, 25
Gentle stretching, 26
Gluteus maximus, 46
Gluteus medius/minimus, 45
Golf, 98–100
Golfer's elbow, 134–135
Gracilis, 56
Groin strain, 136–137
Growing pains, 15–16
Gymnastics, 100–102

Half-Kneeling Shin Stretch, **60**
Half Lotus Position, 71
Hamstring, 58
Hamstring Stretch
to Bench, **58–59**
harmful, 68
hurdle style, 68
partner-assisted, 74
Hand numbness, 45
Hanging Knee-to-Chest Raise, 187
Hanging Side-Leg Raise with Twist, 187
Harmful movements, 67–74
Headaches, 15, 29, 31, 145–147
Head Stand, 72
Heartburn, 174
Heat therapy, 24–25
Hip bursitis, 138
Hip pain, 54
Hockey, 102–104
Holding, of stretches, 27

Horseback riding, 95–96
Household chores, 159. *See also specific household chores*
indoor, 159–165
outdoor, 166–171
stretching needs for, 11
Hurdle Positions, 69

Ice hockey, 102–104
Iliacus, 50, 55, 56
Infants, 13–15
Infraspinatus, 34
Injuries. *See also specific injuries*
childbirth-related, 13, 14
rehabilitative stretches, 127–149
sports-related (*See under specific sports*)
Inner Ankle Stretch, **60**
Inner Calf Stretch, **61**
Internal abdominal oblique, 55
Internal Rotation Stretch, **35**
Intrinsic range of motion, 75, 76
Isometric Extension, 188

Jaw, 29
Jaw Protrusion Stretch, **29**
Jaw Tuck, **31**
Jobs. *See* Occupations
Joints, 23, 24

Kayaking, 86
Kickboxing, 84–85
Klumpke's palsy, 14
Kneeboarding, 118–120
Knee bursitis, 139
Knee to Chest Stretch, **46**
Knee to Opposite Chest Stretch, **47**

Lacrosse, 102–104
Lateral Neck Flexion, forced, 68
Latissimus dorsi, 35, 36, 45
Laundry, 162
Lawn cutting, 166
Leg
muscles, 59
over head, harmfulness of, 70
pain, 54
Raises, Prone Alternating, 189
stretches, 61
Leg Raises, Prone Alternating, 189
Levator scapulae, 30, 32, 34, 35, 45
Lifting garbage, 168
Low back
exercises, 184, 188–189
muscles, 45
pain, 15, 54, 141–142, 173
stretches, 46
Lower Chest Stretch, **36**, 38, 40, 41
Lunge Against Wall, **53**, 55, 56
Lying Back Extension, **48**, 55

Lying Cycle Kick, 186
Lying Hamstring Stretch, **58**

Magnesium, 21–22
Martial arts, 104–106
Masseter, 29
Middle Chest Stretch, **38**, 40, 41
Migraine headache, 31, 145
Mopping floors, 165
Morning stretches, 9, 11
Mountain biking, 92–94
Multifidus, 46
Muscles. *See also specific muscles*
    assessment, 23
    cooling down, 9–10
    cramps/spasms, 174
    diet and, 20–21
    irritation/inflammation, 24
    neck, 30
    stiffness, alleviating, 24
    warming up, 9
Muscle tension headache,
    146–147
Musculoskeletal problems, in
    childhood, 15

Nausea, 174
Neck
    harmful stretches for, 68
    injuries, 30
    muscles, 30, 32–33
    stretches, 31, 32
    tension, 174
Neck Extension, extreme, 68
Neck Tilt, **32**
Neck Tilt with Arms Held, **32**,
    34, 45
Neck Tilt with Slight Extension,
    33
Neck Turn, **31**
Nerve irritation/inflammation,
    24
Nose to Knee Stretch, 69
Numbness, 41, 45

Occupations, 150
    bending/lifting, 157–158
    health warning signs for,
    150–151
    sitting, 151–154
    standing, 154–156
    stretching needs for, 10–11
One Leg Stretch, **51**, 56
Open Hand Stretch, **44**
Open Jaw Stretch, **29**
Outer Ankle Stretch, **60**, 62
Outer Calf Stretch, **61**
Overtraining, 75

Pain
    abdominal, 56
    alleviating, 24–25
    exercising and, 25
    "gate" theory of, 25
    growing, 15–16

low back, 15, 54, 141–142,
    173
    rehabilitative stretches for,
    127–149. *See also specific
    pain syndromes*
    shoulder, 132
    shoulder blades, between, 174
    understanding, 24
Painting, 164
Partner-assisted stretches, 74
Patellofemoral disorder,
    139–140
Pectoralis major/minor, 38, 40
Pelvic Raises, 188
Pelvic Tilt, **48**
Peroneus brevis, 62
Peroneus longus, 62
Peroneus tertius, 62
Pike, Inverted and Modified
    Inverted, 70
Piriformis, 46, 50, 58
Piriformis syndrome, 144
Platysma, 32
Post-delivery blues, 11
Posture-related stress, 17
Pregnancy
    exercise/stretching during,
    172–173
    phases, stretches for,
    174–183
    symptoms, 173–174
Prone Alternating Raises, 189
Prone Groin Stretch, **57**
Psoas major/minor, 50, 55, 56

Racquetball, 116–118
Raking, 169
Range of motion, 75–76
Reach Stretch, **37**, 45
Rectus abdominis, 55
Rectus femoris, 50, 56
Rehabilitation, stretches for,
    127–149. *See also under
    specific injuries/pain syn-
    dromes*
Relaxation, 10
Repetitive strain injury,
    148–149, 151
Rhomboids, 30, 32, 34, 35, 45
Riding, equestrian, 95–96
Rock climbing, 87–89
Rotator cuff, 34, 35, 36
Rotator Cuff Stretch, **36**
Rotators, 46
Routines, 63–65
Rowing, 106–108
Rugby, 97–98
Running, 108–110

Sailing, 110–112
Sartorius, 50, 56
Scalene anterior, 33
Scalene medius, 33
Scalene posterior, 33

School supplies, carrying
    properly, 17
Sciatica, 142–143, 173–174
Seated Angled Posture, 72
Seated Hamstring Stretch, **54**, 58
Semimembranosus, 50, 58
Semitendinosus, 50, 58
Seniors, 18–19, 65
Shoulder
    frozen, 133
    muscles, 34, 35, 36, 38
    pain, 132
    pain between, 174
    stretches, 34–40
Shoulder Blade Squeeze, **40**
Shoulder Stand, 70
Shoveling snow, 170
Shower, stretching in, 9, 63–64
Side Lunge, **56**
Side of Leg Stretch, **48–49**, 58
Side Split, 73
Sitting Groin Stretch, **57**
Sitting Lateral Bend, **38**, 46, 55
Sitting occupations, 151–154
Sitting Toe Touch, **51**, 58
Sitting Twist, **49**, 55
Sit-ups, 185–186
Skating, 112–114
Skiing
    alpine/downhill, 77–78
    cross-country, 91–92
    waterskiing, 123–124
Snowboarding, 118–120
Snow shoveling, 170
Soccer, 115–116
Soleus, 58, 61
Spinal Extension, using gravity
    and partner, 74
Spinal Flexion, partner-assisted,
    74
Spinal Hyperextension, lying
    forced, 70
Spine assessment, 23
Splenius capitis, 30
Splenius cervicis, 30
Sports, stretches for, 75–126. *See
    also specific sports*
Squash, 116–118
Squatting Chest Stretch, **39**, 40,
    41
Standing Hip Stretch, **53**, 55, 56
Standing Lateral Bend, **37**, 46,
    55
Standing occupations, 154–156
Standing Shin Stretch, **59**
Standing Twist, **49**, 55
Static stretching, 8
Static work, 10
Sternocleidomastoid muscle, 32
Straight Leg Stretch, **59**, 61
Stress, 11, 17
Stretching. *See also specific
    stretches*
    definition of, 7

goals of, 7–8
    need for, 10–12
    physiological effects of, 7, 8–9
    rules for, 26–27
    vs. exercise, 8
    vs. flexibility, 8
Suboccipitalis, 30
Subscapularis, 35, 36
Sun Salutation Series, Warrior
    Position of, 73
Supine Groin Stretch, **57**
Supraspinatus, 34
Swimming, 120–122

Tall Stretch, **37**, 46, 55
Temporalis, 29
Temporomandibular joint dys-
    function (TMJ), 147–148
Tennis, 116–118
Tennis elbow, 135–136
Tensor fasciae latae, 46, 50, 58
Teres major/minor, 34
Thigh, 56–57
Tibialis anterior, 59
Time
    of day, for stretching, 9–10
    requirements, for stretching
    routines, 11–12
TMJ (temporomandibular joint
    dysfunction), 147–148
Toe Extending, **60**, 61
Toe Flexing, **60**
Toe Touch, **50**, 58
Tooth and head pain, 29
Top of Wrist Stretch, **43**
Torticollis, congenital, 14
Towel-Assisted Stretch, **34**, 41
Towel-Assisted Thigh Stretch, **54**
Trapezius, 30, 34, 35
Traveling, stretches for, 66
Triangle Posture, Revolved, 73
Triceps, 36, 41
T-Stretch, **52**, 55, 56

Unloading, vehicle, 171
Upper Chest Stretch, **39**, 40, 41

Vacuuming, 165
Vehicle unloading, 171
Volleyball, 82–83

Walking, 108–110
Wall Groin Stretch, **57**
Warm-ups, 9, 26, 76
Warrior Position, of Sun
    Salutation Series, 73
Waterskiing, 123–124
Waxing floors, 165
Weight-lifting, 125–126
Window cleaning, 161
Wrist Extension Stretch, **42**, **44**
Wrist Flexion Stretch, **42**, **44**
Wryneck, 14

About the Authors

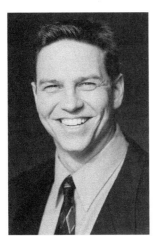

DR. CHRISTOPHER A. OSWALD, born and raised in Stoney Creek, Ontario, is one of the Canadian chiropractic profession's authorities on chiropractic. He has written and spoken on future health-care trends, doctor-patient communication, and stretching. He is a regular author for the Canadian Chiropractic Association's newsletter along with his colleague, Dr. Doug Pooley, President of the Canadian Chiropractic Association. Some of their more renowned articles are: "Philosophy of Chiropractic— Alive and Well in the 21st Century," "The Price of Greatness is Responsibility," and "Communication: The Forgotten Ingredient." Both doctors have a dynamic double-slide presentation entitled "Preparing Chiropractic for a New Millennium" that tours nationwide. The two are recognized television personalities and have represented their profession on several occasions.

Presently, Dr. Oswald owns and operates one of the most successful chiropractic clinics in downtown Toronto. He has helped numerous people find optimal well-being through his innovative approach to pain control and unique use of chiropractic care in conjunction with stretching. Among his patients are nationally ranked athletes, leading Canadian performers and musicians, and some of Toronto's most successful businesspeople.

During the last 7 years, Dr. Oswald has lectured to numerous organizations on stretching, exercise, and assuming responsibility for one's own health. The more notable of his speaking engagements include: the Metro Police Department, Intercontinental Hotels, and the Canadian Memorial Chiropractic College.

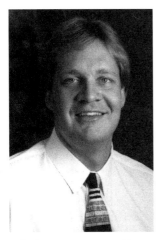

DR. STANLEY N. BACSO was born and raised in Toronto, Ontario. His athletic credentials include competitive football, baseball, and rugby. He was an all-star football player in college and has experience in professional football in Canada. He is still very active in bodybuilding and stretching for maximum performance.

In turn, he has given back to his community by lecturing, motivating, and instructing many young people on stretching, health, and fitness, and how to excel in their own athletic and personal pursuits. He is a staunch advocate of the healthy mind/healthy body concept.

Stan has his bachelor's degree in psychology and social science from the University of Toronto. He specialized for 2 additional years in neurophysiology (cognitive science), and earned his Doctor of Chiropractic degree in 1997 from Parker College of Chiropractic in Dallas, Texas. He is currently completing his post-doctoral diplomat in neurology (DACNB certification).